PREDATORS

TO

COMPETITORS

Notice

This book is intended for reference purposes only; as it will help you make informed choices about your health and lifestyle. This book should not be considered as a substitute for medical advice and everyone should consult with their health care practitioner before making any lifestyle changes.

Mention of specific authors, companies, web sites or organizations does not imply their endorsement of this book.

ISBN 978-0-9878289-0-3

Blunt Force Publishing House

Waterloo, ON

Canada

http://www.blogspot.com/predatorstocompetitors

http://www.facebook.com/pages/predatorstocompetitors

Library and Archives Canada Cataloguing in Publication

Smith, Matt, 1979-
Predators to competitors / Matt Smith.

Includes bibliographical references.
ISBN 978-0-9878289-0-3

1. Health. 2. Physical fitness. 3. Weight loss.
4. Nutrition. I. Title.

RA776.S65 2011 613.7 C2011-907335-8

Preface

I wrote Predators to Competitors because it took me TEN F**king years to not only lose all the weight, but to achieve the physique that I always wanted. TEN YEARS! That's way too long for anyone to endure, and had this book existed then I could have achieved the same 100+ lbs of fat loss in less than half that time! It's the old "Had I known then, what I know now" thing, and it has become both a passion and a chip on my shoulder.

I wrote this book to assemble all the relevant theories, strategies, knowledge and applications that I have found most useful in my journey, and for other average people trying to lose weight or build muscle, or of course, both. I was obese a little more than 10 years ago, clocking in at three hundred pounds! At five foot eleven, that's really heavy! To be clear; I did not diet non-stop for ten years. That'd be bloody insane. Instead, like so many others, I dieted and got frustrated and then tried the next thing. Or I dieted for a while and stalled and decided it was just time to build muscle instead. I lived a continual cycle of successes and failures, and gradual, slow progress. Enough to keep me going, but in hindsight, I realize progress could have come so much faster. Feeling uncomfortable in your own body is a horrible experience, and unfortunately a very common one.

I began my journey lost in the confusion of mainstream diet and exercise advice, feeling very let down by my realization that I'd suddenly gotten way too fat. I say suddenly because I, like so many others, was blind to my weight gain. I avoided the scale at all cost. I skipped every trip to the beach for years. I would duck outside at the mere mention of a camera or group photo. Looking back I was in blissful denial, not ignorance, as I clearly did not want to be seen in that condition. It was just easier to ignore it than to come to terms with the body within which I was not willing to live. I had been an athletic kid, good enough for some football MVP trophies, all-star games and championships, but I always felt kind of chubby. Not fat, just not comfortable or confident in my own skin.

Looking at pictures from my youth, I really wasn't chubby, but when you believe it, it's real. Real or not, it shaped my self concept which was what allowed such rapid weight gain after I gave up football due to injuries. Believing I was overweight made it super easy for my newly sedentary body to pack on the pounds it never could with three nights a week practice, a weekly game and all the other activity of being a kid in the 80's. It was my athletic background and generally good condition growing up that made it so hard to accept that I was becoming fat -- not just chubby, but really, really fat. It was that self-loathing man in the mirror that motivated me everyday while I lost that weight, and everyday since. Although the loathing is gone, the stretch marks won't ever allow me to forget.

My goal here is to put down in one cohesive place everything I wish I knew early on and everything that I have used successfully as a personal trainer. I also hope to shed some light on the billions of mistakes I made and misconceptions I believed along the way. Many of them you yourself have likely made and believed, maybe even today!

Introduction

While I cannot guarantee your success in weight loss, I can guarantee that most of those who read this, if not all, will learn something that will benefit your progress in weight loss, muscle-building and general well-being. Anyone who follows the plan laid out in this book will absolutely change their life. Success comes from the application of the knowledge, not the knowledge per se. *Predators to Competitors* is the culmination of 10 years worth of research, trial and error, heart and soul. Grasp the information, apply it with every fibre of your being and become the predator you were meant to be.

It was when humans manifested destiny by our own invention and control of our environment that we truly became predators. No longer reliant on scavenging for larger predators' kills, we chose our path and dominated our competition. This book aims to achieve the same transformation in each reader. If implemented, the teachings of this book will help reader to become predators atop the food chain, living according to primal instinct and desire, and to become competitors thriving on achieving goals and relentless self-improvement.

As predators we can choose from an endless supply of foods, all of which are easily obtained relative to our ancestors' plights to stay fed. This book will teach you how to harness the power of the predator, using your instincts to eat and to make the most of your meals.

As competitors, we must instill into our minds an uncompromising will to succeed, and to lay rock-solid plans as the bedrock for achievement. This book will help you make attainable goals and give you the competitive edge needed to continually make improvements on yesterday's previous best.

Predators to Competitors will give you the background knowledge to make your own informed choices regarding your health and physique. *This* will give you the framework to create your own life changing plan of attack. *Predators to* Competitors aims to free you from the stranglehold of modern society, to unleash your primal instincts and to fulfill your role among humanity as both a predator and a competitor.

The human animal evolved as a predator, despite lacking many of the natural weapons of the tiger or the sensory powers of the shark. Humans dominated the planet by becoming Apex predators, not by design. We have no claws, nor teeth meant for gashing flesh. We lack the speed of the cheetah and the agility of the falcon. We have no sonar sensory technology in our DNA, nor can we smell a drop of blood in the open water. Instead Humans have evolved as a species by manipulating the world around us which is only possible with imagination and creativity. To become the top of the food chain and to ensure we brought home the bacon, we made weapons to compensate for our short, dull teeth and fingernails. We designed snares, ambushes and other traps to make up for our lack of speed. Predators rely on their instincts to dominate their environment and to ensure their survival. They eat to live, and never graze for the sake of it. Predators eat by their instincts and engage in physical activity only with purpose. Predators in the wild are naturally lean and muscular, though only if their predation is successful. Their success, and therefore their survival, depends on their ability to become competitors.

Competition in the wild is fierce for territory, mating rights, food and survival. Species engage in daily battles within their own pack, and with rivals of their own species. Predators must compete with other species which rely on the same food sources. Humans were definitely the underdogs of the prehistoric competition. Not only did humans have to face off against other near-human species, like Neanderthals who were clearly better built for battle, but also against ridiculous odds like John vs Sabre Tooth Tiger or Jane vs. Mega Bear. Those who cannot compete with their peers either leave in search of an easier life, give up and accept a subservient role, or die in competition. The human predator's greatest weapon is the brain, as we are capable of much more insight, observation and deduction than any other animals with which we had to directly compete. Competitions are rarely won by chance, rather they are the result of planned, precise actions based on sound reasoning and keen observation. Competitors identify the goal and then make strategic moves to accomplish said goal. That is exactly how we switch from Predators to Competitors; planning precise actions based on sound reasoning to accomplish a clearly-defined goal, monitoring the outcome and making adjustments if necessary.

These are the two sides of the human coin that we aim to exploit, by using them as a weapon against fat and illness, and as a tool for building a stronger, healthier body. Being intelligent animals we can harness the intrinsic instincts of the human Predator for intensity, ferocity and drive. By engaging our Competitor instinct, we can ensure that every action is planned, precise and driven by purpose. If you truly want to change your body, your health and your life, you have to attack every day like a Predator, and plan every step like a Competitor.

A Brief History Lesson

ATCG: these letters, representing DNA "bases", repeated in a very specific order of about 3 billion characters, create the blueprint for You: your Genome. 3 billion letters makes a lot of room for variety, and for individuality. That makes three billion opportunities for you to be unique. Three billion is such a large number it's difficult to even comprehend its magnitude. A popular analogy is that the DNA in your Genome (your personal blueprint) if unraveled, could reach the sun and back more than 4 times! Another way to envision it is roughly 200 volumes of about 1,000 pages, the size of a Manhattan Phone book; which would require nine and a half years to read non-stop. Obviously, you are quite unique. Even if you consider yourself ordinary, you are unique. Even if you're an exact duplicate of your twin, you are still unique. Every one of us is a collection of data compiled in this mystic code for construction, function and maintenance; and for mutation and dysfunction.

You see, if you're reading this, I assume you are human. If you're not, rad, I'm not sure how to interpret that, but it's cool. Are you Aliens or super smart terrestrials native to Earth? Hmmmmm. Hope we, the Industrialized didn't screw things up for you as bad as we did for ourselves. Or better yet, hopefully by the time Aliens reach us or the Dogs start reading, we'll have righted the ship so to speak. Humans, you see, evolved from little upright monkey men and in a slow steady progressive fashion, became the planet's so-called dominant species. While equally important to the mechanical adaptations such as our opposable thumbs or upright walking, the biggest leaps in our evolutionary journey happened mostly in our brains.

These big brains are capable of big dreams, revolutionary ideas, care, compassion and love. However, these highly evolved organs also posses the potential for sin: wrath, greed, sloth, pride, lust, envy, and gluttony. The same incredible ability to dream, to think, and to create, built pyramids in Egypt, water ducts in Rome, created beautiful music and art works through the ages and also 24-hour drive-through fast food joints, super-sized value meals and injecting diseases and heavy metals into ourselves. If you're picturing the cartoon devil and angel on your shoulder, you're getting the right idea. You make hundreds if not thousands of decisions, both conscious and subconscious, everyday. Human existence is a complicated juggling act; many of our social norms are there to suppress natural human behaviours. We're forced to fit into a mold we may neither be suited for nor enjoy.

Try to imagine how complicated an animals' life is compared to your own. It's not likely that animals in the wild think about much at all. Perhaps they think about sex during mating season or when Barry White comes on at the Zoo, safety during times of vulnerability and like everything else that is not dead yet, food. It's not very likely that animals think much about food except when they get hungry, and even then it's a pretty simple process compared to that which you and I are accustomed. We have to decide between hundreds of versions of dishes using essentially the same foods and also we live amidst an endless supply of food. An animal on the other hand sees some fruit or leaves that look tasty, and then makes lunch of it. More intelligent animals may have options for food, but they'd be tied mainly to availability, or the effort required obtaining the food source.

Ancient Humans would have been similar: hunting and gathering for sustenance based on what was available in the area during that season. Hunting and gathering was relatively easy when times were good, however humans existed through a whole lot of tough times. Consider, an ice age for example, be it 6 months or 60 years; gathering becomes really hard under a few feet of snow. Hunting was also harder physically, and there were less prey to hunt, so Humans eventually began to prepare. That is, to see into the future enough to know that when snow comes, food is scarce. We started planning ahead based on observation to ensure success; we were becoming Competitors. Competing for survival against the environment and food availability taught us much about planning ahead.

Humankind lived this type of Hunter/Gatherer lifestyle for a long, long time and it's how our genealogy evolved. We, like any other animal, did not evolve in an environment with an abundant, easy to obtain food supply every day of the year. Every species experiences times of food shortage, and in the wild food is much less predictable than it is for our industrialized society - less being the operative word.

The world in which we live operates on waves; times of plenty turn to times of need, hot seasons turn cold. However not much happens overnight on this spinning rock, so between every extreme is a transition; between every peak, a valley. Humans and every other predator on Earth has learned to observe these waves, interact with them, and to follow their lead towards abundant food and restoring vibrant health. Seasonal changes in the tides drastically affect food supply for Predators, and survival for their prey. High tides bring more safety for prey, but low tides make it harder to hide from, and to escape predators. Following the natural waves of the Earth and of the species, predators could gain maximum success with minimal effort. Predators utilize the theory of efficiency whenever possible, expending as little energy as is needed to complete the goal at hand, or paw, I suppose.

As Humankind began to observe and comprehend the annual waves, and to adapt to changes in season and climate, they also transitioned from hunting and gathering to agriculture and the domestication of animals. A few too many lean winters made us decide it was time to take control of our future and to ensure a steady food supply. We started to live out our dreams and create; planting crops so food was easy to find freed up more time to build shelters, methods of transportation, more sophisticated weapons, plots to conquer the world, hitting on cave chicks, etcetera, etc. However, Mankind's conquest of the Earth has come at the cost of the health of our planet and every animal, plant and otherwise living on it. It has also come at the cost of our own health. Cancer, Diabetes, Heart Attacks, Multiple Sclerosis, Lupus, Allergies and Intolerances (and a million other "diseases" of humans, the soil, trees, and animals) are all products of our impact on the environment. Living out of balance with the intended waves has wreaked havoc. My belief is that this is because we, as a species, have strayed from the practices, actions, foods and lifestyles that humans grew up on, in evolutionary terms. We've existed as a species for a long time; we've only been fat, sick, weak and "modernized" for a blink of an eye.

This spinning rock called Earth has been around a really, really long time. It's changed a lot too, and not like the "Wow, you've really grown up since High School" kind of change either. More like a "Wow, you have your arms where your legs were and your head where your right arm was!" kind of change. Yeah, pretty drastic change. Even still, to this day the Earth is changing, whether or not you know it. It makes sense then that beyond the evolution of the planet and its environment, we do not live on the same Earth our Caveman Ancestors did, but equally important is the fact that we do not live the WAY they did. In other words, we do not live in harmony with our evolution. Fake foods, lazy lifestyles, pollution, contaminants, toxins and generally living out of balance with nature have really messed up our species.

By looking backwards we can illuminate the path for a healthy future for humanity; a future wherein everyone acknowledges that he or she is responsible for his or her own health, but also for the health of the planet, and all those around us. As millions wait for science and technology to salvage the health of our species by solving the riddles of our DNA, this book intends to put right what has been wrong for so long. Despite the efforts of our ancestors' traditions, we have lost hold of the healthy balance of living on the Earth. I hope that this information will liberate the reader from the confines of modern society's stranglehold of toxicity and oppression of humanity's natural Predatory instincts.

Radiant Health and a peaceful existence are the intrinsic right of every human on this planet. This book aims to illustrate the evolutionary path of humankind, how we have ended up in such discordance with health, and what each of us can do to restore ourselves to the healthy, glowing, lean, luscious Homo sapiens we were meant to be.

I find it funny that Homo sapiens mean "Wise Man", because modern man is more of a "wise guy". Ladies, don't laugh I mean mankind, all of us. We exhibit behaviours, encourage social norms and consume substances that our families 10 generations back would find ridiculous. To your family of 10,000 years ago, 50,000 years ago, or more, our behaviours and foods would seem completely alien. Driving your car across town to run on a treadmill, for example, would seem ludicrous. Drive-through windows where mountains of food are passed to you, to be eaten while driving your iron beast with wheels. Eating two to three times more than a body needs, while sitting at a desk all day, exerting little more than a coma sufferer, and wondering why said body has gotten so fat and/or so ill. Obesity and disease are so prevalent in society, especially as the body ages, that people accept this as the norm.

It happens to the best of them, others will tell you. Really? The BEST of them? THE BEST of them get fat, sick and miserable? The best of them have trouble sleeping in their soft, warm beds, with a full stomach and no threat from nature? I always found this hard to believe. So I started to read, and to travel, and to enlighten myself on the ways of the world. I began to look to research on remote tribes, or villages outside of industrialized society, where we see men and women in their 70's, 80's and more still in great health, living glorious golden years, compared to our industrialized standard. Clearly they were not living the same lives as we, the industrialized people. They were living the way humankind evolved: in harmony with nature, a body with order and balance.

I recall traveling to The Dominican Republic, visiting a remote village of maybe 200 people; the kind of place you have to take a boat to get to, then cross a bunch of log bridges throughout the various pieces of land along the coast. It was a village in which the people were outnumbered by the livestock. When we reached the shore, we were greeted by our host, and amazed to see a dozen or so dead stingrays in a pile by a few young men with spears. This group looked like an ancient tribe of human predators gathered on the beach surrounding their prey, except for the board shorts noticed on closer inspection. Intrigued, I asked about this group. They were teenagers who had been raised hunting in the ocean for food, and who were so good at it they now made a living out of it. They could stay under the water hunting for so long and because of their extremely physical jobs had absolutely shredded physiques.

Later I met an old man with grey dreadlocks who showed me the shack homes, and cemetery (I asked, it looked so cool. I'm weird, I know). This man, probably in his 80's, has the chiseled physique of an MMA fighter, or a fitness magazine cover model! An old Cover Model, yes. Is there a Geriatrics Fitness Mag yet? Anyway, moving on. More and more of the men and women I met there had this same outstanding physique, and yet, there was no gym in their village. Shocking! There were no protein shakes, no fat burner pills, and no 24 hour gyms for OCD bodybuilders and dieters. Instead, there we homes that needed repairs, animals to tend to and clean up after. And kids, lots and lots of kids. Food growing everywhere, lots of harvesting, lots of manual labour. But above all, there were healthy people. Healthy, happy people living the way mother nature intended. Not a perfect life, nor an easy one, but one in harmony with human evolution.

In the city, where people lived an equally economically tough life, though with many different demands and stresses, I met a young woman working as a waitress. I asked her about life in what appears to tourists as an island paradise, but what in reality has a dark and dangerous side where most of the residents live. She told me of how her mother was sick and she had to work to feed her brothers and sisters. She told me how many of the women she grew up with had left the DR after marrying men they met vacationing there, eventually going to the US, Canada or Europe in hopes of a better life.

In a similarly remote Mexican village I met people who despite living in an equally remote place did not share the same lifestyle as those I'd met in the Dominican Republic. They also did not share the same vibrant health or hardships. This village was remote, but more affluent; not rich by North American standards, but rich compared to the tin shacks. These houses were made of brick, and they were several times the size. A few gardens existed on the larger, hilltop lots, but most of this village was stone, brick and mortar. There was a general store and a few restaurants, even a nightclub, or disco as they referred to it.

The people in this village were not lean or muscular and did not appear to be living a very active lifestyle. A few failed Spanglish conversations left me with more questions than answers, so I went wandering in hopes of finding some of the latter. I found a few English speaking, American Hippies living there who told me that the village was a reserve and could only be inhabited by those born there, or those who marry someone who was born there. The cost of living there was very low as a result, and many of these dudes had decent income, local rental properties and a nice life. One dude, who smelled an awful lot like a Cyprus Hill concert, and still had the ponytail and tie dye, told me that he collects a US disability pension despite living there and lives like a king.

Still not yet satisfied, and a bit bored by my snoozing travel companions, I went walking down a path into the jungle. Smart, right? Well I had a few scary moments like passing a group of horses who had their heels pointed at me, a pack of stray dogs who looked at me like a walking sirloin, and the biggest damn ant I've ever seen! But eventually, between the wild animal scares and ending up dredging through a bird-filled mud pond, I found people! Farmers and Ranchers to be exact, and hard working ones at that. They had the lean, muscular, healthy look of the dreadlocked grand daddy and the stingray hunters of the DR, and that to which humanity is entitled.

I knew then that I was on to something, and that if I could use ancient ways of living adapted to fit into our modern world, I would likely be able to restore my body and my health. I knew I could use where we'd come from to chart my course to where I wanted to be. I knew that the ancient knowledge of our ancestors could outmatch the media hype, commercial brainwashing and marketing madness that was causing so much frustration, confusion and illness.

This fostered an intense interest in me to discover just how humans are meant to live, how we evolved as a species, in hope of finding a way out of the colossal mess we've gotten into with the health of humanity. Along my journey I learned the value of health, and the balance of nature. This is the learning I hope to impart to you.

Going Back; Way Back

Evolution can be a rather hot topic when it crosses paths with someone's beliefs about humanity; especially if those beliefs involve some sort of organized religion. Differences of opinion in the origin of life range from fringe alien ant farm theories, to a higher being and creationism, to scientific coincidence; and EVERYTHING in between. Whichever philosophy strikes a chord with you is just fine, because the origin is simply irrelevant. There is clear, decisive, scientific proof of the evolution of species; including us, and the Earth itself. Many high ranking religious officials have acknowledged this, and just accept it as part of their God's plan. Some scientists believe the Big Bang and the perfect coincidental balance of factors leading to water on our planet are the sole reason we exist. The fact is we're here, we've been here for quite some time and the archaeological record shows us a lot of how we became distinctly human.

The mammalian family tree is very old and very large. It started way back with reptile-like creatures, gradually shifting and changing through various forms somewhat physically familiar to us today (though not the same) and eventually to monkeys and beyond. Though the influences that lead to upright walking, downward sloping noses and hairlessness are not fully known, two general theories tend to arise.

One: as the Earth evolved, lush tropics turned into more open savannas so natural selection favoured a different kind of monkey in that area. Upright walking enabled greater efficacy of traveling long distances, down sloping noses blocked dust better, and hairlessness out of necessity of temperature control.

OR

Two: evolution in and around the water caused hairlessness for swimming, down-sloping noses for diving and upright walking for hunting the waters.

Sea Monkeys, Mermaids, upright monkeys, ancient humans or whatever. I like to call them upright monkey men; the first monkeys who walked upright, and took those first steps away from being just monkeys. The best scientific minds have recreated these dudes from fossils and comparative evaluations with known species. Upright monkey men, while not a very poetic title is just perfect for these little.... dudes and chicks. Being able to walk upright enabled these hairy little pygmies to use their hands more, to hold, to touch, to feel. Their little brains were just fine for their time but would pale in comparison to those reading this work. These little folk weren't particularly bright, but they eked out a nice little monkey life. No shelter building or scrabble; just surviving, foraging and fornicating. Oh baby; a monkey's life!

As the monkey men branched into an evolutionary family tree that more resembles our own, the nervous system, hands and brains became very important traits for natural selection. Brains to come up with ideas, and control of the hands to manipulate the world around them enabled some primitive mastery of their environment. Cracking a nut open with a rock may not seem like much, but this type of Stone Age breakthrough led to new food availability, and better chances of survival, reproduction and prosperity. As we harnessed more food choices, weapons to hunt and fire for cooking, we gradually increased the quantity of calories available for growth. Growth that could be of benefit to our brains, which are much bigger in comparison to our ancestors; our bodies also grew bigger with time as is evidenced by the difference between present day human and the upright monkey men I clearly love to talk about.

Most early tribes were hunters and gatherers; that is, they hunted animals and gathered edible foods. This was an active existence and a full-time job for ancient humans. Gathering required much walking and digging, picking, bending and carrying. Hunting on the other hand required walking or running long distances tracking an animal or herd. A burst of energy was required at the time of the attack with sprinting, throwing, thrusting and an intense adrenaline rush. Whether you belong to the camp that believes the various tasks were divided by gender or the camp that argues division by age or status, the fact is ancient humans had to be active, walked a great deal and exerted themselves thoroughly from time to time. These are clues to how the human body evolved, adapted, and therefore can be maintained.

Periods of food scarcity would have also meant that our ancient ancestors went hungry from time to time. Hunger can be a great motivator; imagine not being allowed to eat breakfast until you showed up at work. You'd probably see fewer people showing up late, especially showing up late with a retail coffee in hand. Stomach growling, no gathered food left, you'd inevitably go find food, or perish. Hunger drives us to do crazy things, like attacking a wooly mammoth. However, when humans realized that a group in cooperation could easily take down a large animal and how much food they could get from one kill, and the frequency of hunting that such a giant beast could provide, the need for better weapons and more advanced preservation was created.

Less energy spent hunting, thanks to technological breakthroughs like bone-tipped spears, again allowed our growing brains to flourish. Techniques like ambushing, and trapping along with keen observation allowed humans to become excellent predators. There's no point stalking a herd that returns to the same waterhole, at the same time everyday. Lie in wait, and attack. A lesson from nature in efficiency. While studying nature and evolution, efficiency was a theme I consistently came across. Natural selection favors traits that increase the odds of survival, and eliminates those that are useless. If it doesn't move you forward, then in perhaps the slightest way it holds you back.

This is the law of natural selection and the evolution of species. Again we can use this information to our modern benefit by looking at evolution as an efficiency machine.

Case in point is the ice fish of Antarctica and Southern South America; a translucent clear fish that has nearly clear blood, leading to the initial, false title of "bloodless" fish. That is not a typo. This small fish, due to the decreasing oxygen content in its home waters over millions of years, dropped the need for hemoglobin to carry oxygen. It is the iron in hemoglobin that turns our blood the dark red sanguine to which we're accustomed. The water there became so oxygen poor, it was easier to absorb through the scales than to use the traditional hemoglobin binding method most of the world uses. So over the course of evolution, as water temperatures dropped in the region therefore decreasing oxygen saturation, so dropped this fish's reliance on hemoglobin. Efficiency at its finest.

Efficiency is a very common theme in evolutionary terms; it is also very common with our own bodies. It is this knack for high efficiency that enabled the Human to populate the entire world. The human body is a wildly adaptable being that can withstand incredible amounts of deprivation. The ability to store extra energy as fat, and then to call on said energy in times of need, was an amazing adaptation for survival. In a time of starvation, a body with more fat stored would stay alive longer than a body in its lean state. So natural selection favoured human genes that enabled mass storage of excess calories in fat cells.

The nutritional status and diet of a pregnant mother influences how much these traits are expressed, in that a well-fed embryo and fetus will be prepared for a world where food is abundant, and storage is less important. Whereas, an embryo and fetus who does not receive adequate nutrition either because of low quality food, or low food quantity, will prepare for a harsh world, where food is scarce or nutrients are hard to come by. In such a scenario the ability to store extra calories would be beneficial.

Those same genetic traits that furthered our ancestors' chances of survival and reproduction, have now got us so far out of control, so out of balance with nature and so sick.

For example the disease Sickle Cell Anemia, a genetic adaptation that helped ancient West Africans survive malaria, now causes severely painful attacks in the descendants of those early malaria survivors. An ill human can still mate, reproduce and continue the human genome; a dead human can not. Therefore nature selected for survival, not long term health. In terms of natural selection, if you create offspring, and raise them to self-sufficiency, you have served your purpose. It is humankind's quest to control all that has lead to our ever-elongating lifespans and the diseases associated with overstaying our welcome, so to speak. Most deaths in our early ancestors were from acute injury or infection. With limited medical resources, a bear attack or infection of a wound from said attack, would often hand the victim a death sentence.

As our ingenuity led to longer lives, we began to see chronic illnesses and the wasting away of industrialized old age. As we outlived attacks of malaria, or cholera, our bodies succumbed to the very abnormalities that saved us initially. We cannot be upset by this genetic hand-me-down, as without it, we would not exist. These abnormalities were needed for our ancestors to live long enough to pass them down to our lineage. Our current obesity epidemic and its related diseases can also be seen through these ancient eyes.

Our bodies are programmed to store excess calories in order to survive starvation. That line is so important, so central to the theme of this book that I'm just going to repeat is again. Our bodies are programmed to store excess calories in order to survive starvation.

I'll scream it one more time for safe measure. OUR BODIES ARE DESIGNED TO STORE EXCESS CALORIES IN ORDER TO SURVIVE STARVATION!

Keep this in mind throughout the rest of this book and it will help you understand the body in which you live. Fat is just f**king awesome in evolutionary terms because it's easy to store and on top of that, humans have a nearly unlimited storage capacity for it. Compared to a few hundred grams of glycogen (stored sugar) capacity, fat is a super advantage when food is scarce. Fat just gets a bad rap nowadays because we don't like how it looks. It does serve both negative and positive purposes, but mainly we just don't like to look at it.

The human body grew up in times of food scarcity and food abundance. In nature there are always seasons with waves of food growing, hatching and being born and therefore humans ate a lot. Contrasted to this time of plenty, were the tough times, when stored food had run out and no new food could be found. It was this continual wave of food that shaped our fat storage ability and current epidemic.

We no longer have to go without food, unless we're in a financial crisis or some self-imposed food restriction. You can decide you want Hagen Daaz at 3 in the morning, and you can easily find it. No doubt that tub of four suggested servings ends up being one, after which our proverbial late night dairy hunter dozes off on the couch. He's not going to burn off those 1200+ calories anytime in the next 8 hours (or however long he sleeps) so it just gets stored as body fat. If he isn't very active the next day, and continues on like this, it's obvious how fat gain takes hold and obesity is the outcome.

Ancient man had no opportunity to get fat, he'd never find enough food without having to expend nearly equal calories in obtaining it, and if by some miracle he did become obese, he's be an easy target for a leaner, meaner predator. He'd be outcompeted by his own peers if not already so by the other species better adapted to the hunt.

As predators by choice and not by design, we humans must use every advantage possible to control our environment, our futures, our health and our destinities. Our capacity for advanced thinking is what allowed us to become predators, and it is also what will return the human race to its predatory right.

Our Family Divided

For some reason after we'd evolved to our current form of Homo sapiens, our population dwindled and a group of our ancestors left Africa. Perhaps in search of food, perhaps to escape drought, perhaps in search of your next American Idol, this group set out on a journey that would eventually lead to populating the entire Earth. The journey as described in *Journey of Man*, by Dr Spencer Wells, is fascinating and very enlightening in that it instills a feeling of human brotherhood. When you look at the journey our ancestors took and the minute changes from one region or country to another, it becomes obvious that we are all brother and sister; we all share the same small family if you trace our roots far enough back. This helps to explain why there are so many familiar faces or voices across all countries; there is likely a shared ancestor. *Journey of Man* helped me see that we are all connected – every person on Earth. As nearly all of us originated from the same small tribe that left Africa (a few stayed behind), we all share some similar genetic traits that dictate what is and is not healthy for us all.

I knew this was relevant, as our genetic make up is nearly identical to their own. We could look to ancient societies and the information and artifacts they left behind, and also at modern day tribes, removed from society who have maintained their traditions. Clearly we have lots in common genetically speaking, being that we evolved from a small group that left East Africa some 50,000 years ago or so, give or take a zebu hunt or two. Yet if you look at the tribe that didn't leave Africa, and who have kept their traditional way of life intact, the San, the similarities in appearance are clear. Many of the features prominent in the surrounding regions are present in these peoples' eyes, skin tone, physique and customs. Their language though is quite different. With clicks, and simple sounds, one can see this as a primitive language, albeit one that was the bedrock for all those that came there after.

Their traditional diet and lifestyle still intact, and unchanged by modernization, includes much fresh fruit and vegetable foods, and lots of hunting. They are fit and healthy, when water and food are plentiful. When it is scarce, life becomes very hard for these modern day Stone Age humans. That may be some insight as to why we humans first left the only home we'd ever known. As humankind travelled up through Africa, the Middle East, Asia, Oceania, Europe, and the Americas over the past 150,000 years we adapted to the new climates with whatever nature necessitated. Changes in skin color due to amount of sun exposure or lack there of, helped these groups absorb the vitamin D they needed. A person living in a northern region required lighter skin that would be super-sensitive to the sun, as exposure was limited. Someone living in an extremely sunny area required a tougher, darker skin to withstand the immense quantity of sunshine inherent to that region. Again it is about balance; enough sun exposure and absorption for Vitamin D production vs. over-exposure to the sun and the damage it causes.

Humankind not only became more physically diverse, we became more culturally diverse as well. Traditions, cuisine, folklore and art all took on the practices and beliefs that were conducive to health and happiness in humankind's new homes. The myriad methods of cooking and preserving foods, all very similar but each slightly unique, provide a great example of a shared wisdom that grew into the practices of each culture.

The spices and ingredients, food combinations and preparation techniques are all traceable in our journey across the Earth. Language too has similarities in the regions in which they originated – similarities which become apparent when one looks at the big picture.

Agriculture is said to have began in the fertile crescent of the Middle East. This is reflected in the many grain-heavy dishes in those diets, and even more so in their lack of intolerances to these grains. Indeed, some wise food preparation practices were likely to originate here too, as they have the most experience raising and eating crops. As we follow humankind further away from its East African origin, the food choices become more and more diverse, depending mostly on geographic location and climate.

Wild rice was eaten heavily near the Great Lakes, where I reside. Therefore it makes sense that even though my ancestors in Scotland may not have eaten it much if at all, if I'm able to digest it well I should include it in my diet, because I am not in Scotland. Fifty percent of my genetic heritage may originate there, but I reside in a different geographic area with its own unique climate and food selection. Asia has a rich history of fermentation in its food, which is clear evidence that they understood the importance of probiotics in their diet. It may also lead to further insight as to why it was so valued there, perhaps due to a deficiency in the soil or local fare not present earlier in our journey. Again it's likely the collective wisdom and the amazing observational power we humans posses. Whether this was brought along during the journey or adapted to upon arrival in a new scene is unclear. What is clear is that humans adapted to new foods they found, and they came up with some damn clever techniques for making some more edible or less toxic.

Where my ancestors lived in Scotland, for example, I found was wet and marshy. Therefore wheat didn't grow well there and oats became the dominant grain choice; this is why Scottish Oatmeal is so popular. It also led me to believe that Scottish people, and their descendants, would likely be intolerant of the gluten found in wheat products. Similar clues into how our ancestors lived in harmony with nature can be found in every country around the world. Trace your family's journey across the Earth and specifically where they settled, how they lived and what they ate. Do this and you will have gained the greatest insight into your own genealogy and how to care for the body in which you reside. The wisdom inherent to each region is a gift from generations long past, guiding future progeny in the maintenance of their bodies and the Earth they'd inherit. The varied diets of the world, from the hot savannas, to the arctic tundra, are maintaining vibrant health for those who follow tradition.

There's not a whole lot in common between a jungle and an ice field, so it should make sense to reason that the foods available in these locations would also be rather different as well. Equally important, the nutrients required for optimal health in those vastly different areas are also vastly different. In *The Jungle Effect*, Daphne Miller writes of her various trips to study the diets native to unique destinations, and the resistance to disease they provide. The Omega 3 fatty acids and the fish that so abundantly supply them are known to fight against mental health problems as well, such as depression, and seasonal affective disorder.

The countries that consume a lot of cold water fish (which have much more Omega 3's), and are therefore likely cold areas, have very low incidence of depression. Taking a cod liver oil supplement during the dark months is one of the keys to learn from this if you reside somewhere that has prolonged dark seasons or you do not get adequate sun exposure.

One the other end of the spectrum, people who live in lush tropics tend to eat less meat and far more plant matter. This is likely because it requires less energy to pluck a fruit from a tree than to hunt an animal in the heat, also because the nutrients required to survive there were provided by the foods available. What is available locally, when it is available or when it has been produced or preserved according to traditional methods, provides the necessities of life.

The heavy use of olive oil and tomatoes in Mediterranean cuisine is another fine example of how each region developed its own food customs based on their heritage and the foods available in that specific locale. For quite a while it was believed that the Mediterranean diet was the healthiest for everyone, because of the low incidence of certain diseases in that region. Turns out, it's not so great for those not originating from there, or at least currently residing there.

Yet again, proof of the importance of locally farmed and produced foods, in harmony with nature, for keeping people well in every place on Earth. So what's in season where you live this week? What grows where you reside, in any given season has the nutrients needed to sustain life in that environment. Clearly then, our food choices shape our futures, our physiques and our health.

Your natural tendencies are likely guided most by your evolutionary background, and this theory has been extrapolated into a practice called Metabolic Typing. An interesting theory and one that fits with the "eat right for your blood type" idea, metabolic typing defines people as Carbohydrate dominant eaters, protein dominant eaters, and mixed eaters. Involving a whopping dose of common sense, Metabolic Typing suggests people identify their type, and eat accordingly. All my research on Metabolic Tying diets led me to believe that I should be following my instincts and eating what my body requires.

The factors that shape our instincts and the food preferences which evolved along with our ancestors are generally varied and related to geographic coordinates. Your genetic material, where it came from, and how it evolved are of equal importance for restoring your health, losing weight and living in harmony with your body.

Genetic Melting Pot

Mankind began, according to our best archaeological evidence, in Africa, and then spread throughout the world. While the route out of Africa may be disputed, in the big picture, it is irrelevant. Almost everyone I've talked to in my research for this book can trace their family back to its country of origin. Sometimes this comes in the less than helpful form of "I'm 1/18th Irish, 5/6th German, 2/3rds Backstreet Boy, 1/100,000,000 Neanderthal, etc. " In many cases, it is only through the names, traditions and artifacts passed down through the generations. This is a big clue, a smoking gun if you will, into your Genetic Dispositions.

If your family lived in a region without a specific food (perhaps wheat) due to its climate (such as wet Scotland), you very well could be intolerant of that food. If your family came from a region with a rich history of animal husbandry and dairy products, you likely fare well on those foods. Safe to say, nobody's tribe evolved on processed foods and a sedentary lifestyle.

My family history is of Mennonite (Pennsylvania Dutch, which came from modern day Germany) and Scottish descent, therefore when I needed help with my own health I began to research these countries' origins, foods, climate, and lifestyles. The Scottish side was pretty easy, as my Grandma came here to Canada directly from Edinburgh and my Grandfather also from Scotland. So it was just researching Scotland and its foods. The Mennonites had a longer journey to study but they still maintain many of their traditional ways of living. Add to this that no one knows all the details of how we inherit genetic traits, so I'd have to watch out for problems in diet and lifestyle from both cultures.

Some of the artifacts, as well, can be very telling. Cook books, for example, are more than a collection of recipes. They are an insight into life at the time of the writing, just as is any written account. Traditions, such as farming, fishing or blacksmithing can be very revealing about the lineage of your DNA and help to provide clues into how you can live in modern society, still in accord with your genetic inheritance. Foods to emphasize, foods to avoid, lifestyle and activity factors, social practices and many more choices you can consciously control will shape how well you fare in health, fitness and happiness. These are just clues though, as life and history offer no absolutes. The fact is, you currently reside in a place that has its own traditions, culture, food and activity preferences. As in every aspect of life, you must find balance.

Using foods that are in accordance with your genetic inheritance, and grown in your local climate is a great start. To understand the importance of eating locally grown food you must look at our species as predators.

As omnivorous (eating plant and flesh food) animals we eat the plants that grow here, the animals that eat those plants, and the bigger animals that eat those animals. The sun, soil and water in the region in which you live, have created plants and animals intended to be healthy in that region. Transplant a Maple Tree into Caribbean soil and it likely won't survive because it requires the nutrients from where it was grown. This is also true of the human body. I've met an incredible number of people born somewhere else in the world, living in Canada and experiencing illness. Invariably it is an imbalance between the nutrients, lifestyle and climate where they originated and those on which they now subsist. The human is a wonderfully adaptable species, however, and has shown to be able to live in every part of the world. Just think, mankind thrives in such dangerous terrain as: jungles, deserts, mountains, arctic tundra and Detroit. It's amazing to think of the varied climates we've conquered and the various foods their inhabitants eat.

Literally, human diets range from purely vegetarian fare, to a diet of only cattle meat, blood, marrow, organs and milk. Not only have we existed on such various diet, humans have thrived on these various diets. An amazing adaptable machine the human body is, if given the opportunity and the necessities of health. Physiologically speaking, we're just animals and should be eating the foods nature intended us to eat. Vegetarian, Vegan and Meatatarian debate aside, Humans evolved healthfully on VERY different diets, depending on geographic location. That should make sense, as the world has many different climates, many different species of plant, animal, fungi and who knows what else we've yet to discover.

So where a Banana heavy diet might be ok in a warm sunny place, eating the foods from that place while living in a cold, dark climate (Canadian Winter, perhaps?) sends the wrong message to your body. If your body thinks it's sunny in Philly, but you're not getting any sun, you're going to soon have problems. Don't jump to the extremist conclusion that you can never eat imported food; just consider their effect on the sodium balance.

If you're not getting enough sun for Vitamin D production, you should be eating meat and/or salting some of your dishes. Switching from Fish oil to Cod Liver Oil would be another helpful addition during the dark and cold months. The key here is the sodium / potassium balance in your blood, and how foods can affect it. In a four season climate, Canadian Mennonites became very proficient at canning and pickling foods, preserving meats, and many other clever ways to make fall's harvest stretch right through until the spring crops arrived. At first I was surprised by the high salt content of many of these foods, aside from the obvious fact that salt is a great preservative. Then I learned of the sodium / potassium balance and its effect on the kidneys, Vitamin D, Calcium, and ultimately our health. Also important is the fact that traditional sea salt was used, not the commercial table salt product which lacks any health benefit. After this I began to connect the dots of local eating and sticking to family traditions.

Picture the foods that grow in each season, and try to pick out their similarities. In the summer, we get lots of fruit and vegetables with high water content; it makes sense as we sweat more in the heat and need to hydrate.

Fall crops are usually tough and need to be cooked, kept well through the season while providing you the necessities of health. The foods specific to a region and a season have the balance of nutrients required to produce health in that region, in that season. Foods in the spring and summer can often be eaten raw and unseasoned. While the sun is abundant, ancient humans would have hunted less in the heat creating a plant-heavy diet in these seasons.

Therefore the kidneys, which store Vitamin D, sense the abundance of potassium from plant foods and don't need to release Vitamin D's more powerful version. The exposure to the sun allows your body to produce a weak form of Vitamin D in the skin. Although it is weak it is still strong enough for the job. Eating out of tune with nature and relying on imported and processed foods causes humans to get sick by messing with the sodium/potassium balance.

In some that may manifest as fat gained, in others perhaps a skin rash. Still others may, due to genetic predisposition, end up far worse off with the debilitating and life-threatening diseases that have become so prevalent in modern societies.

Your body will save the powerful D for when sun exposure is low, as in the fall and winter months. In those seasons, fresh foods are scarce and cooked, seasoned food dominates the diet. Seasoned invariably entails salt, which tips the scale in the favour of sodium over potassium, causing the kidneys to release the powerful form of Vitamin D. It is our relationship to the sun, the life it provides this planet, and us through the plants and animals we eat, that determines *how* we should eat.

If you're extremely concerned about sun exposure's risks, and it does have them nowadays, you still can benefit from some sunlight. Even moderate amounts like 15 minutes can stimulate Vitamin D production and can therefore assist in maintaining your health. There's also balance to be sought in terms of sunlight exposure, in that your body cranks up melanin production when exposed, and melanin has some important functions related to immune function and health.. Melanin is alsowhat gives human skin a darker color, be it a seasonal tan, or the vast differences in skin tone across the globe.

The optic nerve in your eyes also plays into this relationship. There is growing evidence that exposure to bright light upon waking has beneficial effects on human health, and given that ancient man rose with the sun, not the alarm clock, it makes sense that early light exposure upon waking likely triggers some part of our circadian rhythms. While sunscreen can block absorption of sunlight, and therefore affect Vitamin D production, sunglasses can inhibit the production of melanin, which is our natural sun screen.

Again, it's balance; too much sunlight in your eyes can cause serious damage. Just remember that when you're purposely going in the sun for health reasons (or perhaps to get a tan?). Too much? Too little? Too confusing? Just remember to eat by the season. When food is readily available fresh, eat it! When it's getting low, preserve it.

Jam It With Walnuts, Ugly

When humans caught the wave of seasonal shifts, that is to say when we figured out how to tell when seasons were changing we developed ways to preserve the foods we had in abundance. This is yet another example of the ingenious adaptability of the human species, and the reason we thrive in every environment. Nearly all preserved foods have some form of sodium, as does meat. So these tend to dominate the dishes of winter, when all else has run out. They also help us stay in the right seasonal sodium/potassium balance.

Many methods of preserving also include beneficial bacteria; probiotics which proliferate in your large intestine and are necessary for proper digestion and health. Pickled foods, canning, jellies, jerky and other dried foods all kept through winter and kept our ancestors healthy. You can see how traditional ways of living were in accordance with what Mother Nature had planned. Where the foods available did not sustain health, our ancestors found ways to restore balance. Jerky is a great example of how a discovery can become a practice if it is found to be beneficial. A slab of meat left on a rock beside the fire, or out in the sun drying is likely the accident that lead to the invention of jerky. As time went on, dried berries and animal fat was ground into the jerked meats, creating mankind's first portable, and preserved energy bar: pemmican.

Another great example is of the diets of the ancient peoples of Meso America, where some remarkable food practices were created. Treatment of corn with limestone to ward off pellagra and other niacin deficiencies, and the mixing of grains to create whole proteins show off this incredible scientific curiosity and powers of deduction, though they barely begin to scratch the surface. People noticed tribe members getting ill, and that when they changed something in their diet, that person got better. If it did the same for others, and had no ill effect on anyone, it was adopted as a way of life.

In the mid-east, where temperatures can swelter and meats can rot quickly, the use of hot spices was incorporated not just for their flavour, but for their anti-microbial powers. You can find examples of this ancient human genius in every culture, in every region of the earth. Those ways of life are your roots, and you're not very different genetically speaking, from your ancient ancestors. Getting back to YOUR roots is of prime importance as is adapting your modern life to work in harmony with the way your genealogy evolved. You are unique; you are also the only one who can save you.

You are in control of your life and the choices you make everyday. That big brain of yours comes with a lot of freedom, but also a lot of responsibility. In a modern society where we are bombarded with advertising and surrounded by choices it becomes easy to go astray from how your Great x25 Grandparents lived. They lived simply and within their means. They had limited choices for food, so they got creative. We, the industrialized, on the other hand, have incredible variety, mostly of nutrient poor food products. Just look down any isle in the grocery store: so many calories, so much to choose from.....

Fed but never full

At this point I want to reference something I believe is misunderstood, and that is that dieting is inherently unhealthy because it lacks the nutrients needed for health. The "energy" required to keep you alive while dieting to lose fat is different from "nutrition" or what is needed to maintain your health. Many people are eating lots of food, but still lacking in the life promoting nutrients and food based chemicals. The energy, ideally, comes from fat when you're on a diet, but as you'll see in later chapters, there is more to it than this.

Science has allowed us great insight into the human body, so much so that we have pills and potions said to cover all the necessities of life. Entire stores devoted to supplements, extracts and what have you, may be entirely missing the point in health promotion. Imagine that we find out in 50 years that every supplement prior to the discovery of "co-factor importus" was a waste of money. "Co-factor importus" is so damn important that nothing you eat without it can be absorbed and utilized. I made up that name, but the fact is there are probably millions of chemicals and who knows what in the food we eat and we only know some of them. Much like space exploration and the discovery of new animal species, our knowledge of food and phytochemicals, though quite impressive, is still just in its infancy.

The vitamins, minerals, amino acids, and enzymes that can be found in overpriced, overhyped, oversized buckets painted up like the Babylon whore can also be found in much greater abundance in local food, like a modern day masterpiece, painted with a beautiful rainbow of vitamins and minerals, antioxidants and only time will tell what else. They are also much less expensive, and balanced perfectly with nature. Yes, whole foods, those that the Earth intended us to eat and for which to compete for with other animals, insects, bacteria and fungi. All the necessities of life are found in whole foods, and a varied diet following seasonal availability can meet all your nutritional requirements. However, given that the earth no longer resembles that which nature intended for humankind, there is good evidence to suggest that the foods we eat no longer provide enough nutrition to meet our needs.

It helps to clear up the distinction between nutrients and calories, as mainstream thought seems to lump the two together. A calorie is a measure of food energy, as determined by its heat production. A nutrient is a specific chemical needed to sustain life. A good comparison is between a piece of commercial white bread and a slice of homemade whole grain sourdough bread. The white bread is made of more processed wheat and that processing strips nutrients away from the product. In commercial white bread you'll also find a whole host of added ingredients not familiar to most of us, and not so healthy for any of us. The homemade whole grain sourdough on the other hand has minimal processing, has its germ and endosperm intact and therefore many more nutrients, it also has some of the nutrient stealing anti-nutrients deactivated, and beneficial bacteria added by the sourdough fermentation process. Clearly these two have very different nutrient profiles and effects on your health.

Whole grain sourdough bread is full of nutrients and calories whereas white bread has next to no nutritional value, so most of those oddly named ingredients are added back in synthetic form to make it appear like a food product; it has calories but very few nutrients. Thanks in part to these nutritionally heroic traits, sourdough bread has been shown to exert beneficial control on your body's blood sugar balance, throughout the day! Put another way, sourdough toast for breakfast, instead of white toast, will help keep your blood sugar lower for the rest of the day, regardless of what meals follow it!!!

Nutrients are what your body needs and it will force you to continue to eat in hope of obtaining them. If you eat food high in calories, but low in nutrients, you will soon be hungry again. Compare that to a vegetable which has even more nutrients and even less calories, it becomes easy to see how food quality, not just food quantity can affect your weight. Filling up on bread on a daily basis will likely cause you to gain weight. Filling up on vegetables on a daily basis will have the opposite effect. One step further than the nutrient density of vegetables is the nutrient density of sprouts. Sprouts are seeds that have been soaked then rinsed and drained repeatedly. Seeds contain all the nutrients required to provide life and grow a healthy plant, so the nutrient density of seeds alone is immense.

However, as an organism concern with survival, each plant has equipped its seeds with defenses: chemicals to kill, or in our case sicken, the predator of said seed. The age old techniques of sprouting, rinsing and fermentation all accomplish the task of deactivating these defenses. Sprouting however, multiplies the nutrients in the seed on a level unparalleled by any other food type. The abundance of nutrients in foods like these provide the signals your body senses to determine that you're not starving, in fact, you're well fed. My favourite example is of broccoli sprouts, which contain something like 50 times the amount of the cancer fighting antioxidant suphurophane!!!! When you eat broccoli sprouts you can bask in the knowledge that you'd have to eat 50 times as much broccoli to obtain the same amount of nutrients. That's a lot of broccoli; like eating broccoli from morning to night kind of lots. I'll stick with the sprouts, as then I can mix in other varieties of sprouts for their unique benefits.

I like to think of sprouts as my vitamin supplement of choice. A true whole food supplement, not just a pill derived from whole foods, then processed beyond recognition. When you look at their cost, sprouts are king. The amount of seeds required to make a week sized batch of sprouts costs pennies. The true cost is in sprouting them yourself, which is super easy, but obviously not as easy as buying sprouts. However, as you control the sprouts' growth, you can also eat them while they are still growing and alive.

This is yet another benefit to eating sprouts and any raw foods: the live enzymes they provide your body help replenish your own enzyme pool thereby increasing your digestive and metabolic efficiency. It is not just that which you eat, it is that which you absorb. Better digestion leads to better health in every case. Several other means to this end have been discussed previously: however, this deserves review so let's look at how to relieve a digestive system in overload. When you eat a lot of variety of natural foods, especially fruits and vegetables, you ensure a balanced nutrient profile and you're meeting your biochemical needs. There is little to no evidence to illustrate if it is important whether the vitamins and minerals come from plant or synthetic origin, though given our limited understanding of food chemicals I would sway in favour of nature. Sprouts have been eaten by humankind for ages so you can bet they are a healthy and abundant source of nutrition.

Sprouting for yourself is as easy as soaking some seeds, or beans, then rinsing and draining them in an alternating fashion until full growth is achieved, then eating them along the way, as young as one day old. Seeds are dirt cheap compared to commercial sprouts, and your sprouting equipment can be as simplistic as a mason jar, cheesecloth and a rubber band. You can also find sprouting supplies online, where you'll find some really advanced sprouting options to enhance your crop. Ensuring you meet your nutritional needs will go a long way in not only restoring or maintaining your health, they will help you shed weight. When your body senses it has met its nutritional quota, it shuts off hunger signals. This makes it far easier to maintain a caloric restriction therefore causing weight loss. The high nutrient density in sprouts and mature vegetables will keep you full without a lot of calories to store as fat.

When comparing the nutrient data on various sprouts vs commercial multi-vitamins I was surprised to see how little sprouts it takes to match the synthetic pills. Even more expensive multivitamins derived from plant origin pale in comparison. While synthetic vitamins do make a cheap insurance policy against a deficiency, their inclusion to an already nutritionally bountiful diet is the best option. Given the toxic environment we live in, organic foods are a good choice as they contain more nutrients.

However, there are some specific nutrients that could be implemented as beneficial supplements to our diet.

Omega 3 Fatty Acids were a big marketing buzz word for a while and still pop up frequently nowadays. These essential fatty acids (EFAs) cannot be made inside our bodies and therefore must come from our diet. The promotion of fish oil and its many benefits sound like they must be marketing deception. Reduces inflammation. Fights cancer. Protects against cardiovascular disease. Benefits mental health. Stops criminal dead in their tracks and makes them beg mommy for mercy. Ok, maybe I'm getting a bit off track there.

But the fact remains, fish oil, and specifically the eicosapentaenoic acid (EPA) and docosahexaenoic acid (DHA) and other gems we've yet to identify, are real superheroes of nutrients. These nutrients really do it all. In additional to the benefits previously listed, EPA and DHA also help you burn fat. They, and their derivatives, function also as peroxisome proliferator-activated receptor agonists – a nerdy way of saying they can aid the liver in burning more fat, among other things. As if this all wasn't enough, the ladies especially get on board when they hear of the many hair, skin and nail benefits of fish oil. To make sure the homies are on board too, I'm sure to mention that Omega 3 status influences Leucine uptake and therefore muscle building potential.

Dr Udo Erasmus' epic *Fats That Heal, Fats That Kill*, outlines in great detail the healing powers of the Omega 3's, as well as the degenerative forces of the unhealthy, toxic fats. While it is a lengthy and technical read, it is one that is intimately detailed and written by a true expert in his field.

Clearly then it would be wise to increase the intake of these fatty acids by taking a fish oil supplement. However, be wary, as the toxins we've leached into every corner of the globe have affected nearly all the animals, so choose a brand with a proven safety record. Flax seeds and their oil are also beneficial providers of the precursor to DHA/EPA, α-Linolenic acid (A-LNA). So too are chia seeds, hemp seeds, purslane and walnuts. Though the conversion rate in not very effective, percentage ranging in the low single digits, these plant sources do provide many other health benefits.

Flaxseed is purportedly home to a very high lignan content; a chemical that acts like an antioxidant. Dr Johanna Budwig's work fighting cancer in Germany with Flax seed oil and quark (similar to cottage cheese) is proof of the magical powers of these fats and how they can heal the body.

Antioxidants are something akin to firefighters in your body in that they cruise around putting out the fires of inflammation caused by toxins, stress, and even oxygen. Again, it's about balance. Everything in nature has positive and negative aspects: Yin and Yang. You need to breathe oxygen but in doing so create free radicals: little high-speed wrecking balls, which antioxidants can extinguish. Without the negative reactions, we wouldn't exist; we need the balance nature intended in order to maintain the health of our species.

There are tons of different types and sources of antioxidants, and they all have their purpose, and are found in the right balance in nature. An apple for an example of this balance, while containing a ton of beneficial nutrients also contains cyanide in its seed. Odd, right? Why would it need to have a poison in its seed, when a seed's job is to spring new life?

The answer goes back to the explanation of natural defenses of plants vs. their predators. Ancient apple eaters invariably learned not to chew the seeds (bad taste, maybe nausea?) but to just swallow them whole. This way they come out the back end in a not so pretty lil bundle of fertilizer, thus ensuring the continuation of their species and their mutually beneficial relationship with their natural predators.

We humans are likely the only exception to this rule, eventually plucking the seeds so we could plant them where we preferred they grow. However, I wouldn't be very surprised, only impressed, if I heard of primates doing the same.

The entire planet works this way, with mutually beneficial counterparts making life easier or possible, in some cases, for each other. Further examples of natural symbiosis include the feeder fish that remove algae and other hazards from large sea creatures, and parasite-eating birds perched atop their rhinoceros counterpart. Or take, for example, the ever brave blackbird plover, which will sit in the mouth of a crocodile and pick rotting food from between its teeth. Crocodile Dundee gets his dental cleaning, and Dr Plover gets his meal; both benefit so the practice is continued. Should that hungry croc decide to eat his Dental hygienist, then no longer would he have someone removing the rotting meat. This would soon turn to dental health problems and as always, inflammation, then disease. Once balance is lost, so too shall health soon follow.

An imbalance of any sort results in inflammation, and inflammation grows like wildfire. When the body is faced with stress from any source, be it a poor diet, or a saber tooth cat looking to end his diet, it creates an inflammation stress response. Overeating and unnatural foods for example can have this effect, lighting a fire in a very dry forest. Without the food-derived nutrients, including EFAs and antioxidants, among others, the body goes into inflammation overload and some of the result is that toxins are shuttled into fat cells where they can do less damage.

Herein lies a big part of the never ending downward spiral of health; fat causes more inflammation, which can cause..... More fat storage. On and on she goes, inflammation begetting inflammation. We're told that people gain weight as they get older, I guess because we stop playing hide and go seek (?),getting fat and inflamed and just cruising under the medical radar. That is, until overt symptoms begin to appear. Manifesting as any number of clinical diseases, or more accurately, showing enough common traits to be labeled as a specific disease, inflammation is wreaking havoc on our health and health care systems.

The inflammation caused by the host of other offenders humans face such as bacteria, viruses and vaccinations can overwhelm the human immune system and cause havoc anywhere in the body. How this manifests in each person is as unique as the individual, though many similarities usually exist. The manifestation is through the weakest link, or the fastest route to excrete a toxin. The fact is, we are faced with more toxicity every day than our ancient ancestors ever would have in their life span.

Inflammation is not the real culprit here though, just guilty by association. The real problem is that humans are living out of balance with nature, the way we evolved and therefore the way we are meant to live. Our mastery of our environment (including our food supply) has enabled us to live beyond the means for which we were built. The times of famine and short food supply were an integral part of human physiology and maintaining the balance of the seasons: peaks of feasts and valleys of hunger.

The human body was not built to be able to eat as much as is desired, every single day of every single month of every year of a lifespan. When this is permitted, the balance is thrown completely into disarray. Remember that humans evolved through a lot of physical hardship, working hard for the little food we could procure. When our bodies are subjected to an abundance of calorie rich, nutrient poor foods, coupled with a lack of physical activity, obesity and illness are the only possible outcomes.

Amber Waves of Grain

Agriculture dawned a new era in Human evolution, as learning to control food enabled us to increase our population by increasing our food supply. When humans were hunter/gatherers we underwent times of near starvation when food was scarce due to drought, Winter, and competition or otherwise. When the human body gets too starved it shuts down all non-necessary functions, like reproduction. That means more food equals more sex and more babies. Less time spent hunting and gathering makes room for more time working crops and raising kids. Both still physically demanding work that requires many hours of being active.

Abundance of food brought health consequences, true, but it also provided opportunities, as hunter gatherers never had time to, for example, grind wheat and mix it with some other ingredients, wait for it to cook and cool before eating it. The new foods that became available fodder to us such as grains helped sustain us and allowed us to better prepare for tough times. With the same ingenuity that helped us avoid disease, and to store foods over Winter, our ancestors found ways to overcome the health problems associated with the new grains we were eating.

These problems stem from things like enzyme inhibitors and anti-nutrients which are natural defenses of the grain plant. These toxins are intended to keep grain's natural predators, birds and small animals, from eating it. Some animals have the enzymes needed to digest them anyway; humans are not among that group. To humans the effects of these deleterious anti-nutrients were not so immediately obvious, but deadly none the less. So we developed methods of eliminating or reducing these toxins: food practices such as sprouting, rinsing, and fermentation all accomplish this task.

Building societies brought with it division of classes, and food choice would be a prime example of the differences in nutrition levels. We can use this example to help us understand the effect of different grain products, and the concept of "food" vs. "food products". I consider a food product to be something man made, usually lacking in nutrition and loaded with white sugar, white flour, white salt and all the modern preservatives and additives. Back when white bread was a luxury only the wealthy could afford and the poor existed on tough whole grain bread, it was documented that the wealthy began to gain weight (then seen as a status of wealth and status) and to develop diseases uncommon to the labourers and peasants.

Traditional bread making practices eliminated the negative substances while modern practices eliminated many of the healthful nutrients. Lack of nutrients, also known as malnutrition, leads to disease; however there are many ways modern humans are losing nutrients without knowing it and are slowing dying as a result. With time and industrialization, science began to discover the nutrients lost in the processing process, and then to add them back into the processed product. Still to this day, food processors continue to discover nutrients missing in their products and to "fortify" said products with synthetic versions of the nutrients.

Consider the many fortifications of bread, and even more sinister, baby formula. "Humans need more iron"; bam! Iron fortified everything. "Vitamin D is important": Shaka blam! D in everything too. "Omega 3 Superstar"; Whoop there it is. The line between our lack of understanding of nutrients, and the marketing capitalizing on it, has been blurred like a diabetic's vision after birthday cake and beer. The fact remains, we'll continue to discover new nutrients, or the importance of those already known, and then offer a "oops, our bad" along with a new and improved version contains this new priority.

Whole foods, conversely, already contain all the nutrients shouted from the billboards and mentioned above, yet they also contain all the chemicals, nutrients, vitamins, minerals and other worldly yumminess that the universe intended for us to eat.

When you consider that everything in the universe has a shared ancestry, and that everything is built out of recycled stars, it becomes evident that we're intimately tied to this planet, and this planet to its solar system, and so on. Nature has provided life on this planet, and had we not had our multi-million year keg party here, would have maintained health and harmony perfectly. We, like our evolving brains, grew so fast, and we now are dealing with an overpopulated Earth because of our vast expansion and dominance.

We have used our brains to outwit our predators, and have created safety from becoming prey. We've become so successful in competition with nature that more humans die as a result of other humans than of any other predator. Plus, we don't even kill each other for food, or at least not in a literal sense. Then again there have been accounts of cannibalism throughout history so maybe we do to some degree.

Those accounts typically involve far removed tribal situations, or starvation situations such as the Donner Party or Homer Simpson on a Hunger Strike. Starvation can cause people to do some crazy things, as I mentioned already. I think anyone who has tried a low carb diet for a week or more would agree, lack of food drastically changes you.

Consider, however, how many people in your neighbourhood are fed, but deficient in nutrition. You can eat 2000 calories worth of Burger King at every meal, every day – cleary enough to be overfed. Yet in doing this you could still be deficient in a few nutrients, enough to cause problems. Considering how many diseases are linked to a nutrient deficiency, it stands to reason that a low quality diet may be the root of many of today's mental health issues as well.

Omega 3 deficiency has already been implicated in depression, and surely as time passes and science reveals more links of this nature, nutrition-based medicine will be pursued by pharmaceutical producers as it has been by natural food advocates and naturopathic medicine. However, missing the forest for the trees as always, industrialized proficiency will zero in on one or two specific targets and ignore the synergistic balance of nutrients found only in nature.

Rise of the Machines

Industrialization brought about machines to do humankind's jobs on the farms and in the factories, and machines to make cooking and cleaning less laborious. No longer do you need to walk to a safe water station; we'll get it right to your house. Same for food, you can drive to a store that has foods from all over the world, as well as some packaged food that doesn't even resemble those from this world.

You can find a machine to do the work for you in virtually any job. Even war, the cash cow of the industrialized nation, has become more distant, impersonal and devastating. Attacking from further away is safer, and involves more sophisticated, and expensive, weapons. The smart bombers of their day, these behemoth weapons had to be built and sent off to war. Producing weapons, chemicals, and military equipment is big bucks, and the companies that do so are usually affiliated with the government officials responsible for their contracts, although usually well disguised. Likewise, the rebuilding of war-torn regions is big business. Nothing gets a country out of an economic depression better than a war.

The chemicals used in these wars have often been proven to be unsafe to humans too late, as militaries exposed their own soldiers and civilians to them without proving them safe. Many of you reading this have been exposed to these chemicals. However, we were told we needed these chemical weapons to ensure we weren't outmatched by our enemies, who were also developing these weapons.

Money is the bottom line, so anything that can scare or lure people into spending money is good for the economy. Scare tactics, fear mongering, junk science and blatant lies have lead many countries into health crisis. They've led us astray so many times, and for the most part it goes unrecognized or vaguely forgiven. Don't eat red meat, the experts said, it has too much saturated fat. Don't eat butter, same deadly saturated fat; instead eat this weird plastic thing called margarine we created. Never mind that it doesn't taste as good as butter or that it's not proven safe, it's soft at room temperature, and keeps for years on the shelf and in your fridge.

You can't bottle and sell your exercise and lifestyle choices. Same thing for real food; there's no real profit in that. Those foods go bad; we need shelf-safe foods in your home in case there is another world war and food becomes scarce. Let the fear mongering begin. The dominance of food production and profits over food quality and health is probably as old as food itself, or at least as old as trading. But the scale and consequence of the industrial world keeps growing. What was good for the industry is marketed as somehow being better for us, though in fact it is quite the opposite. Even in the face of damning evidence, the food producers and government officials overlook health consequences in the quest for the almighty dollar. As a result, we grow more and more distant from the foods our species evolved on.

In short mankind began to work less for more food, praise wealth instead of health and thus balance was lost. Less walking and fewer bicycles and more automobiles, more restaurants and less farmers' markets, more packaged foods and less home cooked meals. However, Capitalism couldn't stop us there. The consumer was buying, so the producer found ways to make us buy more. Bigger packages, deceptive labeling, inclusion of denser ingredients like high fructose corn syrup and those convenient to shelf life such as trans fats. We kept buying so they kept shoveling more junk onto our plates. They figured out how to sell more calories, less nutrients and more toxins to anyone who would buy it for its perceived value. All wrapped up in a fancy package with a toy for the kids!

Another aspect of human physiology and our evolution that we've lost touch with, moving a lot has been overcome by the invention of the automobile. Don't get me wrong, I love the freedom of having a set of wheels and a tank full of gas. However, I walk or bicycle almost everywhere I go. Cars are great for hauling kids and groceries but when they become your only method of transportation, they've added to the problem. Bicycles have been replaced, but have started to make a resurgence amidst eco consciousness, however e-bikes have now begun to threaten the use of physical energy for transportation yet again.

We will always want more for less, a machine to do every job, a meal cooked in one and a half minutes and we continue to avoid anything that made us work or even wait for our food. The microwave oven is a great example of our use of technology to cure our impatience and indulge our laziness. Invented in the USSR, it became popular the world over and dawned a new market of food products; TV dinners. I've never trusted the microwave. It just seems sinister to "nuke" something you're then going to eat. The fact that the microwave was invented and first banned in the USSR backs up my suspicions with a thread of evidence.

As humans grow lazier, and live more comfortable lives, the industry fills every void in the market place with machines, chemicals and tools to complete our mundane tasks. Gone is the need for elbow grease, as my grandparents would have called it. The industry gives us the convenience we want, and we're paying for it. The way out is not the way through, in this case, it is the way back.

Back to your roots, to a modernized way of living in harmony with your genes and with nature. Back to an active lifestyle, home cooked dinners made with local foods, radiant health, happiness and simplicity. Step back from this industrial machine we live in; to see it from ancient eyes and imagine your ancient ancestors living in perfect balance.

Bigger, Not Better

Everyday your body uses energy to just stay alive, and energy to do things like walking, breathing, backside 540's and the electric bugaloo. The exact number is irrelevant, as it is not static. When you truly understand and accept this truth, managing your body becomes much easier and more intuitive.

If you sleep in, then lay around watching football all day you aren't using very much energy. Compare that to rising early, and playing football all day, where you are clearly using a lot of energy. The difference in energy output, and the amount of food needed to sustain it is obvious, however it can also be very deceiving. We're looking at two individuals on a Sunday; one day of the week. We don't know what the couch-laying, football watching individual has been doing Monday through Saturday. Nor do we know what our football hero has been doing during the work week. Add into this hypothetical comparison that the football watcher is a soldier, and weekend warrior is an accountant. You likely now have a different perception of the equation, as you now have more details and a bigger picture.

The bigger picture is the key; consistently eating more calories than you burn causes your body to store the excess as fat. If you're already overweight you've consistently eaten more calories than you've burned, and this doesn't happen overnight. Gaining weight is a gradual process so sometimes we don't even notice it happening. The scales of health are out of balance, and what's left is a body with too much fat. You have to tip the scale back in the direction of under eating until you restore balance.

This is accomplished by eating fewer calories (not necessarily less food), burning more calories or ideally a combination of both. Diet is by far the most effective method of weight control, or weight loss. However, foods provide us with the nutrients required to sustain health. Therefore eating less than the body requires is inherently deficient in nutrition, which is unhealthy.

Eating enough of the nutrients your body requires, while burning off more energy than that food provides is the ideal situation for fat loss.

The key, again, is balance. Balance between calories in and calories out. Whenever you engage in an activity of any sort you spend more calories than you would just sitting down. Exercise can do amazing things for the human body, especially when combined with a whole foods diet; however most of us can only exercise a few hours per week. While we should strive to increase this amount, only professional athletes have time to train for several hours per day.

Increased Daily Activity is the final piece missing in the trifecta of weight loss. This entails the hundreds of little jobs and activities you go through everyday and again is an area where humans have taken the energetic low road. Stairs or elevators. Bicycle or automobile. Lunch hour walk or feast. Walk in the park or Segway ride? Damn I hate those things.

The small things add up and in the grand scheme, can make quite an impact on your overall health. The human body is simply not designed for 8 straight hours of sitting everyday in addition to its 8 solid hours of sleeping. Even those who work desk jobs have options such as sitting on a stability ball or disk, or better yet a standing work space. You might get weird looks; I do, but who cares? I'm certainly not living to impress others or fit into their mold. Are you?

People who fidget, or tap their feet have been shown to burn more calories than their still-sitting counterparts. The same is true for people who consistently take the stairs instead of the elevator. Standing more often, walking to get files and forms, and just frequently getting up helps make even the most inactive job fit better with human physiologic requirements.

There are a lot of modern conveniences we don't even acknowledge as being options; they are the norm. All the modern conveniences we thoughtlessly employ can be replaced with a more human powered option. In this eco-conscious age, think of using a renewable source, that is your food energy and body fat, instead of some of the less green options of hydro or gasoline.

The standard is for having to move less, so taking this step involves breaking from the status quo and forging your own path through this world. There will be Nay Sayers, there will be obstacles, and there will be rain. Bring an umbrella. At least we have the weather network for guidance, though I've always found looking out the window to be more reliable. Instituting a family walk after dinner is a great start, as is committing to a longer walk for your puppy. Walking or cycling to work is a smart way to save money, fit some exercise in and do your part for Mother Nature by cutting your contribution to pollution and fossil fuel usage.

In my opinion though, nothing beats walking first thing in the morning. In my studies I found many references to long walks in the morning, usually for food or water; but also extending to the movement of military troops. Fare was light to non-existent for these long marches, as walking does not require much energy, and what it does require is easily covered through the use of stored body fat.

Let's Get Physical, Physical

Increasing the amount of daily activity you engage in is a step in the right direction. Notice I wrote activity, not exercise. While I am a big proponent of exercise, I am an equal fan of activity. People tend to associate activity with more enjoyable scenarios: walks in the park, leisurely bike rides with your kids, gardening and whatnot. A lot of what matters in weight loss is consistency over the long term. Sticking with an activity you enjoy is easier than maintaining a regime you loathe. Activity is typically thought of as something you could do several times per week, or even every day, for the rest of your life.

Whereas exercise summons up images of weight lifting, jogging or some form of torturous cardiovascular machinery or worse yet, roid raged body builders, marathoners dropping dead and Richard Simmons sequined tank tops, afro and sweatband. (Shudder)

Everyone is wired and built differently, therefore what constitutes necessity for each is different. Some people are naturally muscular, some naturally thin, so it is reasonable that their exercise program should be different as well. Each of us has an ideal physique in our imaginations, or memories, and that ideal is based on how each of us wants to be perceived. Many of us want to be perceived as not having the weaknesses or imperfections we currently have, so as to live up to our own standards.

Most naturally lean guys have trouble putting on muscle, where as naturally muscular guys tend to put on fat easily. Yet another example of Ying and Yang. A person who wants to look like a runner should run, clearly. They should also look into what other forms of training professional runners utilize. Likewise, if your goal is to look like an MMA fighter, you should mimic their training styles. Utilizing similar training styles, will improve the same energy systems and can have a great impact on developing a similar physique.

However, unless you're a professional, you likely don't have the 8 hours per day to train that the pros do, though implementing a similar training style and nutrition plan will allow you to develop the metabolic pathways these fighters use which have built their bodies beyond average.

All these activities expend more energy than sitting on the couch, so increasing any of them can help you lose fat. However, as you can imagine, there is a fair difference between calories burned during an hour of gardening and an hour of kickboxing.

So while a generally active lifestyle can help lean people maintain their weight, more intense, calorie-demanding activity is required for overweight people to burn fat. Running is often the first choice, probably because of its freedom and anonymity. You don't have to tell anyone you're doing this; in case you fail this saves embarrassment. You also save face by not signing up for a gym membership and quitting. However, running for overweight people can be rather destructive, especially on the knees, ankles, arches of the feet and the spine. Running is not necessary, and not advised for most. It is the energy required to run that is needed, not running per se.

I used running to lose weight initially, but despite a good background of running, the injuries that ended my football career became apparent again; they also became very sore. This was what initially led me to weight lifting, and led me back to martial arts, specifically, kickboxing.

The physical necessities for a predator to competitor transformation as I accomplished, are a dedicated strength training program, a cardiovascular program and an increase in daily activity. Every type of exercise has its pros and cons, so there's no need to concern yourself with which burns more calories, or a larger proportion of calories from fat. What's important is to do what you enjoy, what you can stick with long term and what benefits you the most. Try new things for variety and for the challenge it will provide your body; challenge brings with it the opportunity to improve upon weakness.

However don't confuse variety for stalled progress; many people change their program so often it’s impossible to determine if they've made any progress. In that sort of system, it is unlikely. Programs should be designed for at least 3 weeks, if not three months, and only altered if progress is not happening as expected.

Strength Training refers to any type of training that causes you to apply muscular force against resistance. This could be a weight lifting style routine of barbells and dumbbells, squats, deadlifts, and bench presses. This could also refer to military or gymnastic training where the resistance is your body against gravity. Even yoga and Pilates have a strength training element. As you adapt to the exercise and become proficient at them, you increase your muscle mass and neuro-muscular control. This does not necessarily mean large muscles, that depends on your goals, genetics and to be frank, your gender.

I've yet to meet a man who is afraid of putting on muscular size, this phenomenon is almost exclusively female. The fact is women lack the testosterone to build what anyone would consider "big" muscles. Women, who lift heavy weights and are in control of their diets, have the look coveted by the "butts and guts" or "toning" crowds. Lean, athletic and feminine is the result of a properly planned exercise and diet regime for a woman.

The key here in strength and musculature development is progression: continually working harder at pre-determined rates of incremental increases in weight, volume, frequency or speed.

Barbells are the perfect example as you start with an empty bar, and add more weight at each successive workout. Applying continually increasing demand on the muscular system drives adaptations in muscle growth and efficiency, creating a more athletic body.

Multiple progression schemes can be very helpful during times of calorie restriction (aka dieting) as a pure weight increase (single progression) with every workout may be overwhelming to the recovery abilities provided by a limited number of calories. One method is increasing repetition count every workout with an unchanging load, between a pre-determined range (6-12, 2-6, 8-24 depending on goals) and then increasing the load after the high end of the range has been accomplished. Another method would be micro-loading; using smaller than average plates to add a pound, a 1/2 pound or even less, allowing you to add weight at a slow enough rate that a caloric deficit does not inhibit the progression of hypertrophy (muscle growth).

It also feels much easier while dieting, to lift a weight only ½ pound heavier than you lifted at the last session. Mentally and physically, micro-loading can provide a break amidst hard training cycles.

Use it or Lose it

Another key element in addition to muscular development is the message that strength training sends to your body. When dieting, the body looks for the most efficient means of energy, which, oddly enough isn't always fat. In an ideal world, when you go on a diet and your body would use 100% stored body fat. In the real world, it's a lot more complicated than that. Muscle loss can be a real concern and a real problem if strength training is absent in the regime or even if it is performed at too low intensity.

It's the old "use it or lose it" adage in its truest sense, and again a sign of efficiency in the human body. Consistently lifting 500 pounds illustrates the need for muscle and connective tissue capable of lifting 500 pounds. Discontinuing this lifting or lifting significantly less, while in a caloric deficit will result in the efficient practice of shedding the now unnecessary muscle. Muscle is metabolically costly, so if it is not needed, it's gotta go.

I've always thought of all exercise to be the modern day equivalent to our ancient ancestors' hunting efforts. The parallel between strength training and cardiovascular training exists also with gladiators, warriors and athletes. Humans have had to be masters of all domains and our physiology reflects the varied nature of our athletic prowess. Just being fast or just being strong would not have been enough to survive for long in prehistoric times. As predators, humans must train for strength and speed, agility and power. Strength Training specifically I think of as a predation and kill. The intensity, the adrenaline, the physical exertion demanding every ounce of your being, all resemble the efforts of a lion attacking and slaying a zebra.

They stalk their prey, approach in calculated steps and then briefly put every last bit of strength and will into finishing the kill. Finally, they eat until content and then rest, as should be the plan for anyone engaging in physical exertion of this intensity.

The physical competition between two rival male lions or silver back gorillas is a perfect analogy for strength training; brief, ferocious, violent. That is how you attack the weights – like an animal.

I greatly identified with the writing of Arthur Jones, a wild animal trapper and creator of nautilus exercise machines, who studied strength training physiology and likened it to predation in the wild. His idea that we respond to brief, intense movements and lots of rest have also struck me as being in accordance with how our ancestors would have had to exert themselves in the hunt. His High Intensity Training programs were designed to reflect how an animal such as a lion, can build such immense strength and muscularity. Lifting weights can closely mimic the physiological effects of these hunts when the lifter truly applies him or herself and tests their mettle so to speak. However, Jones' main interest was working with bodybuilders seeking the utmost in muscular size; not necessarily my cup of tea.

Being athletic and muscular naturally I've never valued muscular size, but I've always respected strength. It wasn't until I was working out in a commercial gym, home to many steroid using bodybuilders that I began to see the different effect of various training regimes. I recall sitting next to a mammoth of a man, dressed like some 1980's pirate meets bodybuilder, veins screaming steroids on every inch of visible skin, yelling as he grinded through repetition after repetition.

I then grabbed a pair of dumbbells much heavier and performed the same exercise in a quiet, calm demeanor though for about half as many repetitions.

I was looking for a way to develop a lean, muscular and athletic look, not the ripped mammoth look of modern day bodybuilders, so I began to look more into the training methods of my favourite Mixed Martial Arts fighters and NFL players, lightweight power lifters and the strongmen of history. I found that one did not have to have large muscles or bodyweight to display incredible strength. I found records of men at 160 pounds lifting more than I'd seen 300lb Offensive Lineman lifting!

All the information readily available, and being published was aimed again at muscle size and bodybuilding. I sought out information on alternatives to the current wave of bodybuilding propaganda and came across a whole different line of thinking on muscle development.

Predator

Simplicity and brevity were common themes in the early writing of strength training, as also found in the influential writings of Stuart McRobert, including *Brawn and Beyond Brawn.* He preached that reduced overall volume and exercise inclusion made for not only more focused, more intense workouts but also increased recovery.

His detailed descriptions of the lessons he learned in the weight room echoed many of my own and his disdain for steroid use also aligned with my opposition. His dogged gospel of perfect technique over weight or ego, while initially met with stubborn denial, proved to be incredibly beneficial for imbalances in posture and strength development.

Less important than the chosen rep ranges are the chosen exercises, with compound barbell, dumbbell or body weight exercises topping the list. The big, basic moves like deadlifts, squats, bench and overhead presses, chin ups and rows, have worked for millions of people for decades. As my interests grew more and more toward lifting very heavy weights, I found my body changing faster and faster. Every leap in weight lifted corresponded with an equally impressive loss of fat and change in physique.

Learn proper form, start with a light weight and consistently add more weight in progressive increments and/or complete more repetitions. Repetition ranges effect the body on a linear scale from pure strength in the 1-3 range, through strength/hypertrophy in the 4-6 range, to hypertrophy (muscle growth) in the 7-12 range, and endurance above 12 reps.

I've always preferred low repetitions in the 3-6 range, and this has been echoed by many of the people I've been fortunate enough to work with. The intensity you can apply to such short sets is amazing and will greatly enhance your results. The lowered volume also provides a break for your recovery systems, as mentioned, a definite benefit while dieting. I found the justification for this in the writings of Pavel Tsatsouline, specifically his *Power to the People*, and *the Naked Warrior*.

The type of muscular growth induced by this type of work builds dense, strong, rock hard muscle; this is known as myofibrilar hypertrophy. It is primarily growth of the actual muscle fibers, creating thicker, more tightly compacted muscle with great strength. This type of training generally causes less soreness, therefore easier recovery.

On the other hand hypertrophy work induces more sarcoplasmic muscle growth, which is muscle cell growth and has more of an effect on muscle size and less so on strength. This is bodybuilding style weight lifting which is associated with more burning sensation (caused by lactic acid buildup) in the muscle and more pump afterwards. This style is important as well as it can increase blood flow and therefore nutrient transport, capillary density and many others.

One thing worth mentioning is the role lactic acid is believed to play in the increase of growth hormone associated with strength training. In essence, the lactic acid produced in body building style training triggers an increased surge of a hormone responsible for a plethora of beneficial effects.

So many in fact it's been compared to a hormone version of the fountain of youth. The burning sensation you feel when lifting weights for high reps? That's lactic acid. The key is to push through that pain and get more reps, essentially until you can complete no more. So even within the narrow scope of strength training, there is great variety in styles as well as outcomes. How much of each depends on your goals of course. Utilizing all the repetition and weight parameters allows you to meet your full potential, and therefore should at least be explored as an option.

Macro cycling between strength and hypertrophy with sweater and beach season, respectively, is a popular approach. Mini cycles of several weeks or months are another. Another method I've employed with great success is to include several repetition ranges into the same workout session aka wave loading. As always, balance is the key, so find what works for you.

Keep in mind that it is wise to work fom all the angles, so as to best reach your full potential. Starting each exercise off in a strength range of 1-6, lowering the weight and hitting the hypertrophy range of 8-12, lowering the weight again and going for broke on endurance in the 16+ range in each workout is a brutal but effective technique to accomplish this goal.

Here you're stressing the muscle with a high percentage of your maximum endurance, then pushing into higher rep ranges which increases blood flow, thus speeding recovery.

Competitor

Predation is a great metaphor for lifting weights and its likeness can help illustrate the intensity required in the weight room. However, for the most part, in a hunt the prey just wants to escape the predator; he does not intend to kill the predator and then take all his belongings including his family.

Only mankind had the devilishly big brains coupled with the physical might for that type of plunder, and in times of need attacking another tribe for their food supply was not only the quickest route to dinner, in could be the only route.

Daily competition for mating rights or Alpha Male status, food or territory has shaped the human genome's competitor instinct. Therefore, mankind had to be able to fight, to run great distances and to outlast his competition. We needed to be as strong and ferocious as the lion, but we needed to be swift like the leopard and endure at high intensity like the albatross.

Mankind would also need Cardiovascular Training to fully conquer the planet, and the competitors that sought to conquer us. Cardiovascular Training entails any type of training you can sustain for longer periods of time that also challenges your breathing and increases your heart rate. Running, cycling, boxing, skipping, dancing and anything else that can work up a sweat all fit the bill for cardiovascular training.

Progression is again the key here, as you must continue to push harder, move faster and last longer in order to force adaptations from your body. The concept of exercise progression is far more important than it is made out to be by mainstream gyms and the health industry. For your body to continue to make adaptations to exercise, you must continually give it new stimuli to which to adapt.

After years of no exercise, a run around the block will elicit an adaptation, however after a few separate runs around the block, your body will have adapted; it will be easier to run that block. However, if the run stays the same, so does the body. Add another block to the run and your body has to adapt. Run that block faster, and your body has to adapt. The same is true of every form of exercise: you need greater resistance, repetitions or speed. This is again linked to efficiency; your body will adapt only the amount truly necessary and will lose this adaptation if it is deemed superfluous.

At some point, some exercisers will reach their genetic potential, or perhaps just their desired level of strength and conditioning, health and physique. To stay in the same shape is known as maintenance, where the individual seeks to only maintain their current state, not to improve it.

It takes less to maintain strength than it does to develop it; roughly 1/3 the amount. This standard can be used to bolster the effect of a fat loss diet, freeing up more time for more metabolically costly exercise, like cardio training.

One of the main complaints when dieting, obviously enough, is hunger. We're hard wired to get food at any cost when our bodies sense starvation, though this response is partially learned and can be trained. When your body is training too hard and has limited recovery ability from the calorie restricted diet, hunger becomes a major concern.

Abbreviating your strength training regime into maintenance mode, using a cut of up to 2/3 of either volume or frequency, can allow your body to recover better and decrease the hunger response.

Staying in maintenance for strength and focusing on more calorie consuming exercises (such as running, boxing, swimming) can kick a stalled fat loss attempt in the rear and into high gear. I liken "metabolic" style training to the chasing of a herd in ancient hunts, or to the battles mankind faced with ourselves and with all around us.

Martial Arts and all of the fighting sports draw clear connections to battles of ancient times so it's easy to see how they fit in with the genetic lineage from which we derived. Running also has its obvious uses in prehistoric times, so it's yet another favoured exercise. However, prolonged running of great distances would have been used sparingly if at all. The human body is obviously more adept at sprint style running than marathon style.

For proof, take the example of the 1st ever marathoner in ancient Rome, who dies at the end of his journey. Why we created a sport based on that, I'll never understand. For further proof, look at the physiques of the marathoners from your country of origin.

There are some very fit looking Kenyan marathoners, but most everyone else looks like shit. They look drained, scrawny, wrinkled, and generally like death warmed over. Yes, there are some who stay fit through the addition of strength training or some other form of muscle maintenance, but they are the exception, not the norm.

Swimming, rowing, climbing and even long distance walking are all activities humankind has engaged in for millennia and which can have a profound impact on your health. These activities are so varied in their metabolic demand that no clear conclusions can be drawn about the eating that preceded or followed these activities historically.

In modern times, this will come down to preferences for the most part; if you suck at tennis when you haven't eaten yet, or get your ass handed to you in Judo when you're hungry, you should probably eat beforehand. The more energy demanding the activity, the more important pre and post workout eating becomes.

What modern knowledge has given us is the understanding that pre and post workout nutrition can drastically affect what physiological changes will occur. It makes sense that providing energy around times of high energy use and adding nutritional building blocks around times of building would enable more intensity and efficient construction.

Likewise it seems like common sense that eating a lot during times of inactivity would enable rapid weight gain.

This is the basis for nutrient partitioning; the idea that things we do, lifestyle and food choice affect what our bodies do with the calories we eat.

Partitioning, again

In its purest form, nutrient partitioning in practice is to eat most of your calories around your activity. The activity both uses the food to fuel movement and increases the uptake of the nutrients, allowing less to be shuttled into fat cells.

Just as diabetics are told to exercise before eating to aid in nutrient uptake in the absence of insulin (using instead something called GLUT-4 receptors) and to burn off excess glucose in the blood, these practices employ nutrient partitioning. GLUT-4's are glucose transport proteins that are not dependant on insulin. GLUT-4 receptors are what we're exploiting if we consume carbs and protein before and during exercise. They help get more glucose into the working muscles to prolong activity and assist with added intensity.

Glucose, derived from carbs, is a preferred fuel source, and exclusion of carbs shifts your metabolism towards fat burning. By decreasing or eliminating carbohydrates, glucose's stored form, glycogen, will be used up, and then the body shifts over 2-3 days into a state called ketosis.

Working on a sliding scale in reference to how low carb the diet is, ketones will be created to fuel the brain and any other glucose dependencies. In its extremist form, it's known at a ketogenic diet; named after the ketones, which is a glucose replacement product we create.

Due to the fat loss benefits of short term carbohydrate restriction and the benefits of carbohydrate intake before and after glycogen burning exercise, a more sophisticated approach can be added. Said concept would be more efficient nutrient timing.

Nutrient Timing refers to eating most if not all of your starches and sugars, pre and post workout only. The rest of the time, you essentially eat a low carb diet, which allows some additional fat to be used as fuel over a standard diet. The glycogen draining nature of weight training, fasting, and/or low carb dieting creates space for the incoming carbs to be preferentially stored.

The human body can only store upwards of 500 g of glycogen in the muscles and liver, depending on the size of the individual. Based on this, there are various methods to accomplish this depletion/supercompensation cycle. Low carb diets can accomplish this over a week or more, less time is needed if exercise is added. Fasting during the morning hours accomplishes this too, though to a lesser degree, more frequently. Whichever system works for you, right now, is the best.

They all come down to carb restriction except pre and post workout, and basing more calories around times of need. If all you've done is walk and sleep, maybe even sleepwalk, you don't need much food. If you've lifted weights for an hour, sprinted on the track, and did kickboxing sparring for an hour, you're gonna need to eat a fair bit.

As every human's physiology is unique, so too are the reactions to these factors. However, exercise has been shown to increase nutrient uptake into muscle over fat, so eating after activity is obviously beneficial. Equally important is what you've eaten before exercise.

Some people feel fine exercising while fasted, however, everyone can benefit from some implementation of a proper pre-workout nutrition regime for its proven improvements in performance, recovery and strength. The absolute minimum is to consume protein, or even better Branched Chain Amino Acids (BCAA) prior to any intense exercise.

Inadequate protein intake prior to intense exercise increases the breakdown of body protein, which is not desirable at first glance for those trying to lose fat or improve their physique. BCAA specifically can help limit breakdown, and to increase protein synthesis (building) all in a low calorie package.

Consuming the moderate sized meal 2-3 hours before a workout is an excellent plan. This gives enough time for most meals to be digested, and assimilated so you'll be prepared for your workout. Follow this with a small snack of quickly digested fruit and nuts or juice/Gatorade and whey, 30 minutes before exercise to get some nutrients circulating in your blood stream.

As mentioned, some folks feel fine exercising with nothing but protein beforehand and there is some evidence that this can improve some markers of fat loss and muscle building, increasing the results expected beyond what can be explained by calories alone. The theory is that the fasted training creates a bigger disruption to homeostasis, resulting in a larger adaptation.

However, compliance is king, so if fasted exercise necessitates a lower training intensity or decreased recovery, then it should be eliminated. In that case pre-workout nutrition should be strictly enforced to ensure top notch training on a consistent basis.

These nutrients will be utilized for fuel or aid in recovery as blood engorges in the working muscles. Eating after your workout provides the building blocks of life so your body can repair the damage you've caused by making yourself stronger and more fit.

Glycogen is most efficient shuttled into muscle from starchy sources, such as bread, oatmeal and potatoes. In addition to this, a small amount of fructose should be included as it is preferentially stored in the liver, returning the body to an anabolic state. The feeding after training should be the largest and most carbohydrate rich meal of the day.

Of course adequate protein should also accompany the post workout meal to provide the amino acids needed for building muscle. Just as your body is trained in a circadian rhythm, it can also be trained to store more calories in muscle over fat and you can also rewire your hunger response.

Ghrelin is a hormone intimately tied into your hunger, and it operates on a learned daily curve. The times of day that you're accustomed to eating trigger a hunger response.

When you force your body to override these signals and forge a new meal pattern your Ghrelin pattern will soon follow. Start only eating at noon and you'll soon only be hungry at noon.

After sleeping for the night the human body has used up most of its circulating nutrients and some of its stored sugar (the preferred fuel), so when your body calls for energy to power low intensity activity like walking, body fat is readily called upon to do the job.

Any excess calories stored after last night's post-hunt feast will be used up in today's long walk. We can mimic this by incorporating some type of low intensity exercise on a daily basis first thing in the morning, or as early as the individual can tolerate.

Breakfast after this type of activity is optional and dependent on how it affects your energy levels and recovery, and depending on if you are trying to lose weight. If you feel sore and tired from not eating after this, then you should be eating afterwards. If not, the option is entirely related to your own preferences and appetite. Prolonging the fast until lunch or later is a great strategy for burning more fat, benefitting insulin sensitivity and increasing nutrient partitioning.

When to Work Out; The Great Debate

While the main component of effective exercise is consistency, there is enough evidence to support the efficacy of proper exercise staging, or how you sequence your workouts. This is thanks to developments in sport science, and the clearer understanding of the energy system it has provided.

Recall that glycogen is the primary fuel used by your body to produce movement. Exercise of a moderate to intense nature draws upon those glycogen stores, so when one has completed some form of glycogen burning exercise, adding some form of lower intensity exercise can greatly enhance the efficacy of the workout. A cool down period appropriate to the workout can be thought of as a cleanup for any leftover fuel circulating in your blood.

This was the standard practice in the gym where I began training, whether or not anyone knew it. The weight room was upstairs and the cardio machines on the main level. So inevitably, we'd start downstairs to warm up, head upstairs to lift weights, take our time coming back down the stairs on wobbly legs to finish off with a brief cardio session.

Lyle McDonald's incredible book *The Stubborn Fat Solution* details a method of staging an intense but brief workout session followed by a few minutes rest and then moderate cardiovascular work.

This works on a similar principle of spill over and clean up, though in this case the spill is initiated specifically for the cleanup. It can be very effective to follow any intense exercise by a brief rest and some lower intensity work, though it may take some getting used to if you currently finish with a short and easy cool down.

Again, following the yin and yang of your body's circadian rhythm you can place certain types of exercise in your routine according to the energy they demand. If you cannot give your all to intense exercise in the early morning, then you should perform those activities later in the day when you've had some food for energy.

You still can likely take a walk in the morning, and follow this up with your normal breakfast routine. Any exercise will help you make the most of the food you eat, so even this seemingly easy walk is a great practice to incorporate. The more movement the greater the metabolic rate, and more effective nutrient partitioning.

Taken to the extreme this can be seen as eating and performing like an athlete: eat, train, eat, train, eat, train, eat, sleep, repeat. You can see why athletes have little problem with excess body fat, at least those whose sport or position do not benefit from the added weight.

Every time this above proverbial athlete eats, he/she is either fueling a workout, recovering from one, or both. If said athlete is eating primarily whole foods in harmony with their genes and environment, body fat will be somewhere between a non-issue and non-existent.

Those whose job does not entail 8 hour days of exercise and eating (napping too!) can still find ways of mimicking their ancestral lifestyle, and exploiting the above mentioned metabolic boost and nutrient partitioning effects. Already mentioned is low to moderate exercise in the morning either on an empty stomach (if tolerable) or after some light food for fuel (dates and milk perhaps); this will burn up any circulating fuel left over from the overnight fast if nothing is eaten before; either way, it is a boost to the metabolism early in the day, setting up a fat burning environment during the AM hours.

Continuing the fast after the workout is permissible, but may or may not be beneficial. Your body will continue to run on body fat after the workout whether you eat or not, as some studies have recently shown. Therefore eating after the workout may enhance recovery and this would help keep cortisol levels down.

On the other hand, eating after low to moderate intensity may not be necessary as the recovery demands are low, and in this case, keeping the body fasted may be of benefit to overall weight loss. This is especially true if followed by the upcoming recommendations.

Another exercise session or walk around noon hour before the lunch meal will set the stage for moving from the catabolic AM to the anabolic PM. If the midday session is scheduled to be intense, it may be preceded by a small meal if needed, or performed fasted (with BCAAs) if tolerable.

The benefits of pre-workout simple carbs and quickly digestible proteins have been proven and discussed already, so the reader can be informed and make their own decisions.

Those who feel they lose muscle when dieting may benefit more from pre/post workout nutrition than those who retain muscle mass naturally or are at their ideal body proportions and not trying to increase size.

In either case, eating something after intense exercise is a practice everyone should incorporate if possible. This shifts the body towards recovery, repair and building of tissues after a morning of breaking down body fat for fuel.

The midday workout may not be possible or preferable for all either; in this case an intense workout prior to dinner makes more sense. The key is to stage the majority of your calories around intense workouts which require them to either fuel movement or recovery.

When your body is constantly busy with working on repair and building there is little left for fat storage, especially if the fuel is coming from whole foods which are not preferentially stored as fat anyway.

Once the midday exercise has been completed, the pre/post workout meals shift the body into anabolic mode and the Parasympathetic Nervous System now dominates the AM's Sympathetic Nervous System. Rest and digest are the priorities of the evening hours, which most people find fits naturally with their energy levels.

I have never liked eating breakfast (maybe brunch instead) and don't find I get hungry until dinner most days. I live a very active lifestyle which has its own appetite suppression, however part of my preference for AM fasting is practical. I bicycle to work, so carrying a bunch of food can be a pain in the.... Back, to be honest.

There was a time I biked to work with at least 15 lbs of food, ceramic containers, drinks, powders and potions, on top of the necessary business casual attire. That made for uncomfortable transportation; it also made commuting much harder. However, I'd fallen prey to the brainwashing of the supplement pushers and mainstream fitness. I HAD to carry all that food and BS with me every day or I'd lose my hard earned muscle mass or absolutely destroy my metabolism. Total BS. I was working against my natural instincts, and felt like I was banging my head off the wall, month after month.

Working with your body's tendencies is much easier, and more efficient, than fighting against them. Less activity and more food throughout the evening primes the body to recuperate from the day's rigors.

Feasting, resting and sleeping provide the building blocks, energy and environment to create a stronger leaner body. Most of the repair is done while you are sleeping, so making special considerations for sleep is important too.

Last Train to Sleepy Town, USA

All too often those struggling with weight issues overlook the importance of sleep, and given that the majority of adults nationwide are sleep deprived, problems with sleep are common. Eight hours is the recommendation, but for every doctor that espouses this standard you can find someone who claims to run optimally on six, seven, ten, twenty four.

The fact is everybody is different, as is every day. If you ran for eight hours your recovery needs are going to be drastically different than if you watched TV for eight hours, so clearly not only does your nutrition vary, so too does your need for sleep.

Ingrained in your body's circadian rhythm is your genetic standard for sleep, which will change according to a great number of variables. The primary release of growth hormone is during sleep, and given the anti-aging, fat burning and muscle building properties of growth hormone, you clearly want to get all you naturally can. You should be going to sleep when tired and waking naturally, and the changing season's sunrise and sunset times will greatly affect your sleep patterns and needs.

If you set the tone for good sleep and can rise without an alarm, then your body is getting adequate sleep. In some instances, setting the tone is the most important part. Just as it is vital to set the mood in the bedroom for romance, setting the mood for sleep can also pay dividends to your health and happiness. It's no more difficult than initiating the sexy mood with a little Marvin Gaye and scented candles.

Humans would have always slept according to their circadian rhythms, falling asleep after the sun sets, and rising with it. When the world gets dark, we sleep; even the ever present fire only provides a dim light.

There would have been no televisions or late night internet forum arguments to stir the emotions and keep one awake.

Therefore avoid any mentally or emotionally charging stimulation in the evening as much as possible, perhaps opting for a light hearted comedy over a "this could happen to YOU!" type expose. Reading, meditation and other soothing activities can help saturate the brain with positive chemicals, helping to induce a drowsy state.

Bright lights before bed are unnatural and can mess with some people's ability to fall or stay asleep. The use of candles or night lights can keep your toes from continual pain, while getting ready for bed. Some people will find that they do not require much light at all to function.

This can be explained partially through two mechanisms, only one of which we can control. That which we can not control is genetic, and includes among other factors, the ratio of rods to cones in the human visual system.

As color vision grew, nocturnal vision subsided, therefore those with color blindness (such as myself) likely see better in the dark than our full color vision counter parts. The factor we can control, somewhat at least, is memory. Pay attention to the route you take each night dressing, brushing your teeth, locking doors, etc, and soon you will have a visual representation of the layout imprinted in your memory. What may seem like a hassle at first can help improve your sleep drastically.

In the bedroom there should be few distractions, and a simple, clean decor to soothe the soul and cleanse the mind. Sounds from nature, such as rain, waterfalls or oceans, can help put you into a deep relaxation and kick start the sleep and recovery process.

A soothing audioscape can also help block out disrupting noises like neighbors, traffic, or howling cats at 4 am. The room you sleep in should be free from light so as to not interfere with natural sleep cycles, and you should take steps to ensure a solid night of sleep.

If you wake to urinate often, cutting back on evening liquids may be in order. If you wake with some other sort of issue (breathing, digestion, mental stress) professional help should be sought immediately. Many health problems can be expected if a good night's sleep is a rarity.

Luckily in Part II of *Predators to Competitors*, where we begin to implement the program and discuss each step in closer detail, a program for sleep enhancement will be laid out for you. While it still involves some work on your part, the majority of what needs to be done will happen automatically and you will once again be able to wake up naturally, feeling refreshed and alive!

The Need to Feed

Food is a necessity, but when survival is prominent in your concerns, being exposed to predators is a liability. So ancient humans developed the ability to withstand great physical demand without any food, and we still carry this in our genome today. Periods of up to 72 hours without food have been shown in studies to induce no negative health impact and can contribute a large quantity to a weekly calorie deficit, not to mention its improvements on blood parameters.

Though most people I've worked with fare better on a 16-24 fast basis, up to 72 is possible, not necessarily advisable. Some people just can't seem to go without food for any period longer than their average break between meals. There may be some type of blood sugar fluctuation involved, or just a susceptibility to the hunger related hormones. It would have been a liability in ancient times; being so hungry stuck in the tribe's cave, as a saber tooth cat stalks outside hoping to make lunch of you. You would try to break your fast but end up becoming Hello Kitty breakfast.

Luckily, most of us don't have those types of stressors in our modern lives, so food availability begins when you wake up, and ends when you sleep. For some crazy bodybuilders, or sleep eaters, it literally never stops. Unfortunately, this is not how humankind evolved, and much of our digestive and obesity related suffering can be attributed to this imbalance with our physiology.

Our physiology developed over the span of millions of years; wherein foods were plentiful at times and scarce at other times. A perpetual tug of war between feast and famine shaped our genes and we must restore this balance to find order in ourselves.

Consider the aforementioned tribal situation, wherein we find our Stone Age stars stuck in a cave, hungry, being stalked by an equally hungry saber tooth cat.

Well, a few options present themselves; a) try to outsmart the tiger and go for a dinoburger, b) wait out Tony the tiger and hope he doesn't come in looking for a sit down meal, c) eat one of your pals, or d) starve.

Whatever the conclusion of this tale brings, the inevitable end is that our caveman ancestors ate eventually. They were probably pretty damn hungry and went to town on whatever they happened to find or kill.

The period of fasting allows the body to use its stored fuel, and to clear out any old toxins and junk from their stone age trunks. Your trunk too, though not so antiquated, could benefit from some junk removal. Even if your trunk is a mini, smart or otherwise small metaphorical vehicle's storage space, it too could use some old fashion spring cleaning.

No Need to Feed

Nearly every major religion has some form of fasting incorporated into its yearly calendar of festivities. Muslim Ramadan, Christian lent, Buddhist Monks, Mormons, Hindus and countless more all practice some form of fasting.

Ramadan is a month long fast of daily restriction from dawn to dusk. Christianity's Day of Atonement, a 24 hour fast. Buddhist Monks often fast from noon until the next morning, as a practice of discipline and for its health benefits.

Fasting is a very simple method of accomplishing calorie restriction, in that not eating for one day of the week decreases your food intake by about 14%. Conversely, you could cut your daily food intake by 1/3 by just skipping a meal.

Take into consideration that most diet recommendations use a 10-20% deficit, and you see that fasting can be an easy means of accomplishing this. Weight loss or management is one clear benefit here, but add to that increased lifespan, reduced chance of cancer, cardiovascular disease, immune disorders, diabetes and a slew of other ailments.

Improvements in blood lipid profiles can also be expected; which means not only can you cut your food bill by about 14%, if you're taking high blood pressure or other medications, you might be able to cut that cost too.

The importance of meal frequency was pushed to the mainstream for years; eat small meals every 2-3 hours, nibbling away like a god damned hamster or your muscles will literally fall right off, or worse yet your "metabolism" will come to a crashing halt. Bullshit. What might be good for the industry again pushed to the masses.

When you're eating every 120 minutes you have to be prepared with your meal replacement shakes, protein bars, Tupperware and the whole entourage. That's money, baby.

Who makes money off of fasting? A few books have been written on the subject, some scientists have studied it, that's all I can think of. There's no fasting industry. What would they sell? Count down meal timers? "Three, two, one; EAT!" Perhaps T-shirts with clever slogans like "I'm fasting. Fuck off".

Fasting inherently entails avoiding the consumption of any food product, and you can't sell a void as far as I know. Maybe Brittney Spears and Hollywood can, but as far as a product that will secure repeat customers and garner profits, fasting is a bust.

Bling, Bling

Fitness itself is a business now, with specialized high tech fabrics that wick sweat, advanced running shoes with bubbles, cylinders or tubes, and billions of dollars of exercise equipment.

To keep exercise clubs spending is the trick; clubs buy a bunch of machines that have a long life, so in order to make them spend more money, the fitness industry continues to come up with newer, "better" machines designed to appear high tech. Clubs will buy them because their customers want them, thanks mostly to their slick advertising, with ridiculous statements like "burn 300% more calories". More than what? Eating a turkey sandwich?

Again, it's all about the benjamins, Puff. If you buy a $30 pair of running shoes and hit the pavement everyday, you are not part of the machine! The industry wants to convince you that you need their machines because there is little profit to be made from self sufficient exercisers.

Electrolyte replacements, pre-workout glucose gels, micro fiber towels, run designed water bottles, and so on. Do you need these things? The magazines sure make it seem like you do.

Ask yourself if these things were needed for our ancestors to achieve health, strength or a lean body.

Given the advertising in popular health magazines, you'd think a creatine deficiency was the reason for so many people's struggle to build muscle or a caffeine deficiency responsible for so many fat loss failures.

Perhaps acai berry from who the hell knows where is the answer to our health problems and obesity; perhaps Santa Claus will bring you some at Christmas if you're good.

If there's profit to be made, the product exists; if the desperation exists, a product will fill the void. Everyone is looking for an easy solution, and the industry knows it. You'll be told just what you wanted to hear, but hey, the placebo effect is real, so at very least you'll get some benefit out of it.

While there are supplements that can help your fitness goals, the fact is that most of the supplements available are garbage. They're either mixed with fillers and minute amounts of the effective ingredients, or they're based on unproven ingredients and marketing hype.

Nothing can beat old fashioned hard work and discipline. Nothing is cheaper yet harder to come by. Nothing produces results like applying yourself fully and gritting through the discomfort or deprivation. Seeing the body you've always wanted appearing in the mirror due to nothing but your own determination is a remarkable experience and the only way to ensure you get healthy, not just fit.

Quick fixes do not become lifestyle choices, and fasting is easy to incorporate into your own routine. It also replaces obsessive compulsive dieting behaviour, calorie counting or what have you.

Fasting combined with exercise can have some interesting implications, and my reviews of ancient lifestyles seemed to indicate that much activity would have had to have been done in fasted conditions. These avenues lead me to Martin Berkham's Lean Gains website and protocol.

Hands down, the expert on exercise and fasting, Martin's research seemed to validate every theory I had or exercise practice I'd been testing. However, although Martin takes it a few steps beyond, and has a more stringent protocol than I, his methods were very similar to my own and would entail the same nutrient partitioning effect.

Anyone interested in the health benefits of fasting and especially the relationship between fasting and exercise should check the resources at the end of this book for the Lean Gains info.

You could, and I have, spent hours on his website reading free articles. The dude is a genius, and apparently a master of cheesecake. His inspiration has created quite a few high protein cheesecake recipes in my kitchen!

The only significant difference between our approaches is that he maintains a set feeding fasting schedule and always schedules eating in the afternoon to evening window (even if exercising in the am), whereas I maintain my clients schedule most of their calories around their workouts and implement occasional 24-48 hour fasts, especially for those who cannot do daily AM fasting.

The fact is exercise science has shown the benefits of pre and post workout nutrition, so they should be included to ensure the utmost performance. When on a calorie restricted diet, much of the day's calories are the pre and post workout meals. For many, too much food pre-workout can negatively affect training, hence the recommendation by Martin and myself, to add BCAAs pre-workout, or at least some protein to limit bodily protein breakdown.

I feel the rest is dependent on the individual's needs and preferences. True, there may be some physiological benefit to training fasted, though it is greatly outweighed by the importance of intense training. On the other side, the individual may train first thing in the morning which excludes the option of eating a full meal beforehand.

Said individual would benefit from BCAAs pre-workout, or by eating dates with some whey protein upon waking; because dates are nearly pure glucose, they provide instant energy and whey is the quickest digesting of the majority of proteins. A few dates with a handful of nuts makes a great homemade energy bar.

This is quickly digested and won't sit in your gut while you train, where it would engorge your stomach with the blood your working muscles require. This snack could perhaps be eaten alongside a caffeine containing drink like coffee, or better yet green tea, full of antioxidants and other awesome phytochemicals.

Better still, green tea with lemon, which potentiates the beneficial qualities of green tea with its high vitamin content.

The caffeine initiates the hormonal response of adrenaline; this releases chemical messengers that bind to receptors in a lock and key fashion, thus releasing more energy. The epinephrine and norepinephrine released from this fight or flight response can be harnessed to jump start a workout with intensity.

Fasted or not the key is intensity, so if you find you can maintain intense workouts while fasted then do so. However if you find that your workouts suffer when you are less than fed, then clearly should you choose to implement fasting, you'll also need to use caution in implementing an effective workout nutrition program as well.

Fasting on non-training days, with only low intensity activity is an effective method many employ with great success. With a few weeks under your belt, you'll likely start to become hungrier on training days, post workout, and much less hungry on rest days.

Again, this is training your body for a new normal. The old normal clearly hasn't been working perfectly, or you'd likely not have bought this book. Training your eating habits helps to train your hunger hormones and allows you better control over your appetite.

After a few months of implementing fasting for weight loss, you will find your groove and your hunger during fasts will virtually disappear. When trouble arises during a fast, or more accurately, when hunger arises, filling your stomach with water is a great solution.

Most importantly though, fasting is an easy means to a healthy end. When dieting, the calorie restriction necessitates small meal size, which may not be fulfilling to some. By not eating breakfast (oh the heresy) you can spread those calories across the next two meals making them larger and more satisfying which helps in adherence to the diet.

Adherence to the diet is the prime concern for fat loss success and health restoration. If you can't sustain the changes for the long term, they cannot exert long term effects. Studies have shown that meal frequency is not relevant, and that the overall calorie balance is the major factor in weight gain, loss or maintenance. For the most part, and aside from the many factors discussed in this book, your body reflects the long term status of how many calories you take in vs. how many you burn.

If restricting yourself everyday with undersized, low calorie meals sounds horrific, then a weekly 24 hour fast may be a better option. Likewise, fasting throughout the morning increases the size of the following meals, which helps keep people full and strict on their diet. If small but frequent meals throughout the week work for you then that is what you should practice. Long term adherence to a healthy diet will bring extraordinary results on the inside and out. If you are overweight you need to implement calorie restriction; that is to say you need to eat fewer calories than you use in order to force your body to utilize stored fat. If you are underweight you need to do the reverse; eat more calories than you expend.

The specifics of this equation (calories in - calories out) are never perfect, as your needs change on a daily, if not hourly basis. However exercise physiology has given us some good formulae to use as a starting place. If they don't work well enough, or too well, you then adjust to find your current numbers.

Roughly 11 calories per pound of body weight is all that is required for you to sit in bed all day and do nothing but breathe. This is obviously affected by the amount someone weighs, so it can be misleading, as fat does not need to be fed, in our case it needs to be shed. Adding weight in the form of muscle can help sway this equation in your favour by allowing you to burn more calories at rest and during activity.

The additional caloric needs of activity vary greatly between individuals, and within each individual's schedule. However, ballpark figures exist as a starting point. The chart below gives these figures:

<u>ACTIVTY COFACTOR</u>

Mostly Sedentary	30%
Active	40%
Very Active	50%

* 30-40 yrs old subtract 5%

So you now have body weight x 11 calories + Activity Cofactor = Maintenance caloric intake.

This number represents the amount of calories you expend in a day, and the amount of food required to maintain your current weight.

As previously mentioned, you have to tip the scale towards caloric deficit in order to lose weight. So a reduction of 10-20% of your maintenance caloric intake might be a good start. Remember that ideally at least some of said reduction would come from caloric expenditure such as increased daily activity and exercise, unless you are already very active.

There's no need to get caught up in the numbers though; I provided them only because some readers will want them. I would if I bought this book; they are helpful if you have no real reference for how much you eat. Monitoring food intake for a few weeks can have a profound impact on your relationship with portion control.

Less food and more activity is a pretty simple prescription to give, but it's damn true. You can find online exercise calculators that will estimate how many calories you burned doing any number of exercises, but again these are only estimates that vary a lot with intensity.

Heart rate monitoring can be helpful to determine what level of effort is required for the different stages of intensity. A more effective and less stressful method is to monitor your weight on a scale and your girth measurements with a measuring tape. Weight and girth going down; doing great! Stalling or gaining weight and girth; cut some calories.

If you're eating healthy whole foods, exercising progressively and seeing drops in both scale weight and girth measurements you are losing weight effectively. If your scale weight isn't moving but you're dropping inches, you're doing fine.

You may just be building muscle while losing fat, or you may be retaining water, which is one of the human body's funny little survival tricks. If neither is happening, you likely need to create a larger caloric deficit.

The Point of No Return

At some physiologic point, which is unique to us all, the pay off of adding exercise while on a diet becomes a pay back. Stress of any kind, including exercise, increases cortisol transiently, and too much cortisol can halt your fat loss efforts dead in their tracks.

So extreme approaches tend to backfire just as much in either direction; too small a deficit to too large. Consider it an evolutionary insurance plan, if you diet and/or exercise too hard, you will buckle and binge eat. We're wired that way so we don't starve. As always, the key is balance and finding what is right for you, right now. However we can use the knowledge of this emergency survival plan to our advantage, in that we have some great evidence as to what happens in severe diet conditions.

The Minnesota Starvation Experiment was conducted in 1945 to determine the most efficient means of starving and refeeding (eating more than "usual") prisoners of war. They essentially put these men on diets equivalent to modern day extreme diets (around 800-1200 calories/day) and monitored what happened to their weight.

Long story short, they lost weight in a linear fashion, predictably and as expected, for quite a while and then got stuck. Despite the rather extreme caloric deficit, their weight loss slowed dramatically.

A mid way reward was implemented and the men were allowed to eat as much as they wanted that night. Many of the men woke up to urinate in the night, more frequently than usual. All the men woke up the next day several pounds lighter.

This is what is known as a whoosh in modern day weight loss lingo. The best explanation yet has come from one of my absolute favourite writers, Lyle McDonald, more accurately, from one of his former professors.

The idea is that the body holds on to water in the fat depleted cells during times of extreme weight loss, and eventually this water is lost in a mass dump. The water may just be enough to keep the cell alive or to maintain body weight homeostasis.

Another genius survival mechanism of the human body perhaps, though not every one is susceptible to stalls and whooshes. Some folk can lose weight in a linear fashion for quite some time, others will continue to stall and whoosh repeatedly.

I have consistently found women to be very susceptible to these phenomena and that their monthly water fluctuations further complicate the matter. Girls are just whacky is what I usually tell them.

The whooshing likely has two components to its physiology some of which we can influence for our own benefit: water loss and water uptake. First we'll address the actual loss of water. Water loss can be affected by inducing sweat, diuretics or fluid restriction.

When the human body has been starving, or dieting/exercising too hard, weight loss will plateau as cortisol rises. The stress on the body due to limited food for fuel or bodily maintenance, and heavy amounts of work cause a stall in the expected weight loss pattern.

Further dietary restriction or added exercise volume have no effect of breaking the plateau, therefore it's clear our anti-survival mechanisms are at work. This is a big piece of the weight loss failure puzzle, wherein newcomers to weight loss experience some results initially, stall and then give up altogether out of frustration.

On the other side of the equation, and often handed a bum deal, is water uptake, or retention. Water uptake can be affected by exercise, diet and sodium loading; however the location of said water can have a profound impact on your physique. The fact is that water under the skin looks bloated and fatty.

Water inside a muscle cell, however, makes the muscle appear larger and fuller. Remember this, as it will be important when I tie all this together. For a minute, let's return to our archetypical dieter, who has lost some weight initially and now has stalled. This is the fortune of nearly all who engage in weight loss the conventional way; depressing, really.

But wait; what's that in the sky? A bird? A Plane? No. It's a flying potato!!! Our hero, Starch! Increasing the amount of calories you eat, especially starchy carbohydrates, periodically can break this weight loss plateau while also allowing the dieter to enjoy the foods they've had to eliminate or restrict in order to drop weight.

This is thanks to a small link in our carbohydrate digestion chain, called the Hexosamine Metabolic Pathway. Picture several large tubes headed downwards and a small horizontal tube linking two of them. Housed in this small tube is a metabolic sensor that detects how much carbohydrates are being eaten and turned into glucose.

When carbs are depleted through diet and/or exercise the body will attempt to stall your weight loss efforts, but when carbs are increased, the sensor sends the message that you're not starving; you've once again found food.

This allows the anti-starvation mechanisms to ease off so further weight loss can resume; the body senses sufficient food supply, therefore storage becomes less of a pressing issue. Caveman Dan outlasted the Saber Tooth that was outside the cave and he found the jackpot of potato patches. All is well, the human race will survive.

The Hexosamine sensor has some effect on the hormone leptin, which is correlated with body weight and has further effect on overall weight loss. An average person on an average diet would have an average leptin count, barring some genetic defect of course.

A lean person on a diet trying to get leaner will have very low leptin levels. The heavier the person, the higher the leptin level. Obese people have sky high leptin levels, so higher is not necessarily better. There may be a physiologic limit to leptin levels, or perhaps, similar to insulin resistance (Type II Diabetes), the obese become resistant to leptin's effect.

Since leptin injections, back to normal levels, can rejuvenate the dieter's metabolic rate, restore hormonal balance, and enable further weight loss in the lean, striving for balance is the secret.

Bringing lean dieters above normal leptin levels does no more than normal levels. Perhaps anything above normal levels of leptin are superfluous; likely is the possibility that obese folks become desensitized to leptin's effects, so it loses its power much like insulin in a diabetic.

Or that we're just really good, genetically speaking, at storing fat and not so great at getting rid of it.

Interrupting your diet periodically is known as a refeed, or carbing up, and can be very beneficial, more so the leaner you are. Each person reacts differently, so start out with moderate sized carbohydrate refeed and test how much you find right for you.

As mentioned already the upper limit to glycogen storage is 500g, less for smaller individuals. One would think that 500g of carbohydrate would be the limit, and for some it may be, however for those who are exercising intensely upwards of 1000g could be incorporated into a refeed without any de novo lipogenesis (storing carbs as fat).

During a refeed, weight gain is expected although only temporarily, due to glycogen storage in muscle which requires three times as much water for its storage. You should look leaner after a refeed though, as water will be pulled from beneath the skin and shuttled into muscle cells. This comes back to the water gain side of the aforementioned equation. If glycogen is depleted enough, the water that could be lost as a whoosh would theoretically be taken up into muscle along with glycogen.

Water Wait

This is part of the water uptake side of the equation; both carbohydrate and sodium require at least three times as much water for their storage. So water is pulled from elsewhere, and diverted into the muscle cells, both making them look fuller and increasing their fuel storage capabilities.

Dry carb refeeds, where less than average liquids are ingested, can be especially effective at pulling water from underneath the skin creating a very lean look. This has implications for appearance enhancement for a beach trip or a hot date; it's not necessarily more effective in terms of actual fat loss.

Alcohol has also been implicated in the whoosh scenario, in that it is a powerful diuretic and when preceded by a carbohydrate refeed, can initiate some rapid water loss. I have found herbal diuretics, as well as saunas, and sauna suits to be useful as well in instigating an overnight dump of water.

I believe it has to do with interfering with some sensor or mechanism in the body that regulates water retention in times of weight loss stalls. Any type of forced water loss or restriction can be dangerous, and requires the user to take caution and not cause themselves harm. This is likely tied into leptin and its effect on body weight set point: the weight your body is comfortable operating at.

However, the water loss involved in a whoosh does not appear to carry any negative consequences and it may be a necessary component of weight loss for some people.

Lean dieters reaching extreme leanness require a refeed physiologically, and everyone can benefit from them psychologically. The frequency and duration of the refeed are dependent on the dieter's goals, current body fat and muscle make up, among many other things.

When fat loss is the goal, and there's a lot of it to lose, err on the side of refeeds that are less frequent and smaller in nature, then adjust upwards to find your optimal refeed strategy.

Starchy carbohydrates are preferred by muscle, whereas fruit sugars are the choice of the liver. So when refeeding, a small amount of fruit and or other sugars are acceptable to refill liver glycogen and switch the body into anabolic (building) mode from catabolic (breaking down).

The majority of the carbohydrates eaten during a refeed should be of the starchy variety, such as breads, potatoes, rice, corn and cereals. If you feel you need to eat the foods you know you shouldn't, this is the time, as you'll have already employed some damage control.

High fat, high sugar treats are usually the go to for deprived dieters. There is some evidence that this system, called "junk loading" can be quite effective in physique enhancement in that intramuscular triglycerides (fat stored in muscle) can be replaced similarly to glycogen.

Weekday dieting with weekend refeeds are a natural system for most, however many struggle with limiting the refeed when it happens across a weekend. In this case a weekly 24 hour refeed might be best. Perhaps the gung ho method of 12 days of straight deprivation followed by a weekend of overeating better suits your needs. However you choose them, refeeds are fun and they help your body burn more fat in the long run.

As already mentioned the frequency of refeeding is dependent on many factors, such as how well weight loss is occurring, how deprived the dieter feels and amount of fat the dieter is carrying.

High levels of fat correlate to high leptin levels, so the physiological need of a refeed is greatly reduced. However, for most people dieting just plain sucks. No one really enjoys depriving themselves of the foods they love; if they do, they are sick and should seek help.

So for someone with 50, 75, 100 or more pounds to lose, refeeds are more of a psychological break from dieting. They still may prove to have some physiological benefit in the obese as well, as these mechanisms are not well understood yet. However in this instance, with much weight to lose, a smaller refeed would be a better choice. At least one meal, and at most 5 hour refeeds work great for those with a lot of weight to lose.

The leaner you are the larger and more frequent these refeeds should be. There are numerous implementations of this approach, ranging from extreme 10-12 days of deprivation to 2-3 days refeeding, to more moderate approaches such as refeeding on carbohydrates only after weight lifting workouts, when nutrient partitioning is at its peak.

This is known as an every other day (EOD) approach to refeeding, if workouts are staged every other day. Otherwise it's more like a cyclical diet strategy, which may or may not be associated with ketogenesis; which is the state of extreme carbohydrate deprivation.

A method I've employed with great ease and success is what I call cyclical circadian dieting (CCD); fasting or eating light morning to noon while doing low intensity cardio and eating pre and post workout only. This provides great balance as you can use primarily fat for fuel in the morning, and then switch to anabolic mode for the evening and its more intense exercise.

CCD employs the same physiological tricks as more extreme, prolonged approaches but the dieter never goes too long without food making it great for long term adherence. Weekly variance can be employed by eating at or above maintenance on weight lifting days, and fasting or eating lighter on rest days.

Using the aforementioned 2/3rds principle of muscle maintenance, one could schedule less frequent but equally intense weight lifting sessions interspersed with several days of low calories or fasting.

For heavier folk trying to lean out, smaller and more infrequent refeeds work better, more psychologically than anything. This is because leptin has been found to be produced in a number of different human tissues, including fat cells.

As fat cells themselves produce much of the body's leptin it's obvious that fewer fat cells will produce less overall leptin. However the story is more complicated than that. This is because leptin is not only tied in to your body fat, but body weight sensory systems too.

Your body seeks efficiency which usually means maintaining the status quo, which just means that your body likes you just how you are. Sounds sweet, poetic and a little romantic. Wrong! Not so sweet when your brain doesn't much care for your body's appearance in the mirror.

Leptin is likely tied into the mechanisms our bodies use to determine if we're losing weight. Stalls are likely a result of the body trying to maintain its set point; the weight that it currently find most efficient.

Set points are tough to break and your body will fight hard to maintain the weight at which it is currently most comfortable.

I have found that we can use the body’s stubbornness about body weight set point to our advantage; once you understand the problem, the solution usually becomes quite obvious. While those seeking to lose a lot of weight will just need to grind it out through set point stalls, leaner folks can exploit them. This is accomplished by dieting to, or just below the set point and when the body weight begins to creep back up, a more anabolic approach is implemented for a few weeks, allowing the return to set point to be fulfilled by muscle growth and glycogen storage, instead of fat regain.

With determination and the use of leptin boosting carbohydrate refeeds, a new set point can be established. However most experts believe this could take several years at a decreased body weight. This is also a piece of the weight loss failure puzzle so common today.

I believe this set point theory can be used to explain some of the efficacy of body recomposition; building muscle and burning body fat simultaneously, at least within a given day/week/month.

Allowing the body to retain its set point weight, but changing the ratio of muscle to fat, may be a more plausible method than extreme cutting and bulking cycles. To some, this is known as "culking" and can be a great alternative to getting fat and sloppy in the offseason.

As your body changes and adapts to the new exercise stimuli and your reduced body weight, you too must adapt the plan that brought about these changes. As your body becomes lighter it requires fewer calories, as well it burns fewer calories during activity and rest compared to its former heavier version.

So the diet and exercise program that worked initially must continually be updated to spur progress forward; further reductions in calories and further increases in activity.

Progression, in every sense of your plan, is of prime importance to achieving your ideal physique.

Cut the Crap, Jack

Fasting, as previously stated allows time for internal spring cleaning, also known as detoxification. Most of you will have seen those late night infomercials for some detox product where they provide the disgusting figure of 5 pounds or more of fecal matter stuck to your colon causing your "pooch" belly.

If you never saw it, welcome to the grossed out club. This is but one of many signs of an overloaded digestion system. Gas, bloating, indigestion and heartburn are a few more warning signs.

When humans continually shovel in food faster than their body can digest it, the system gets backed up like a really stinky rush hour traffic jam.

Continuous eating not only slows digestive efficiency, it has the potential for even more danger. When the food doesn't move through your system fast enough it begins to rot, which is to say it is being eaten by bacteria inside you.

There are billions of bacteria living inside each of us, and it's the amount and ratio of beneficial to destructive bacteria that affects your health. At this point, probiotics have become a household name, and a marketing ploy aimed at the health conscious consumer. Probiotics are the good bacteria, and there is a lot of variety in the population of these "good guys" in each person.

The problem arises when the "bad guys" take over and start eating all the food that's sitting in your intestines. Problems with the sodium/potassium balance already discussed, cause spill over of the harmful bacteria from their home in the large intestine into the small intestine and stomach. When they get out of their poopy large intestinal jail cell, they throw a party, raid the refrigerator and make a major MESS!

This robs you of the nutrients you need, and it allows these harmful bacteria to flourish, upsetting the balance within you. As they flourish they continue to feast on your dinner and they begin to release their own toxins into your digestive upset.

Those toxins overload the natural detoxification system of the liver, kidneys and lymph, and ultimately lead to diseases of many different faces and symptoms. Just as each of us is unique, so is our reaction to toxic exposures and stress; when the system is overloaded the symptoms show up in the weakest link or where there is genetic predisposition. The root cause is always an overburdened body out of balance with nature.

The immune system can either become so overwhelmed it can not keep up, or in some it can go postal destroying everything in sight including valuable muscle or nerve tissue.

Thus is immune disorder. When you take into account the awful amount of toxins to which we're exposed everyday, you can see how our bodies just can't keep up if we're constantly overburdening them.

Toxic Shock, Baby

Pesticides and herbicides are on our food, even more heavily so on imported food, where our competitors have a longer opportunity to feast. Chlorine is in our drinking water, which destroys beneficial bacteria in our bodies.

Fluoride is in the water with its uncertainties and implications on health. We're injected with vaccines and the unsafe preservatives some of them entail. We're exposed to smoke from factories and exhaust fumes from cars. There are hormones in your meat. There's electromagnetic poison coming from your TV. It's Toxic Waste and it's all around us.

When the body heals itself through detoxification and through weight loss, many toxic substances will be traveling through the body. It is a wise practice to take steps to ensure the utmost removal of these toxins, and this is a lesson I learned the hard way, and which I've witnessed in others as well. For some it can be weakness or sore joints, for others perhaps hair or skin problems.

When the body is gaining weight in the form of stored fat, typically there are toxins abound in the diet and environment; most fat-gaining diets are heavy in processed and junk foods, and as mentioned, we're surrounded by toxicity. Also I say fat-gaining diets are toxic with great certainty because it's hard to get fat eating organic fruit, vegetables, meat, nuts and seeds; they fill you up too fast.

One of the easiest neutralization tactics we have is to stuff the toxins into fat cells or clump them to the wall somewhere in the digestive system. When we go about removing these toxins they can cause havoc; it really is a demoralizing blow, as it comes while the individual is feeling positive about what they've accomplished FOR their health, only to be back handed with some sort of problem.

Many don't see the connection to weight loss and detox, so they assume what they're doing must be harming them. The burden is on the owner of the body to determine what is truly best, and what is truly harmful.

Sweat is a great excretory route for toxins, and this has been known for centuries. Most ancient societies that had cold seasons employed some sort of sweat inducing sauna ritual. The health benefits of saunas and sweating in general have been verified by science; as usual, we have proven what our ancestors already knew to be fact.

Sweat inducing exercise, or activity of any sort should be incorporated. If you're the type who never sweats, you can seek out pore opening creams or the use of vinyl sauna suits, or neoprene clothing, all of which can help induce a good sweat.

Water is another important issue when detoxing, as urine and feces rely on it and are both excellent toxin removal systems. Your entire body depends on and is made of water, so lots of fresh water throughout the day helps create a fresh body. The more water you drink the more often you'll visit the bathroom, thus providing more opportunity for toxic waste dumps.

Speaking of dumps (haw haw), bowel movements should be regular, hence the term regularity. Most people have a set schedule and deviate only when their diet or daily circumstances differ greatly from their norm.

However if you find yourself to be less than regular, the inside of your body is likely digesting and/or excreting at a less than optimal rate, and some serious clean up may be required.

Dr John Matsen's *Eating Alive* taught me about digestive inflammation and the importance of not over burdening the stomach. His recommendation to not eat, or to eat lightly in the morning sat well with the intermittent fasting regime I had been doing, which at the time was eating lunch through dinner.

He also advised an elimination diet to restore order to the digestive system; removing foods known to be common irritants for a period, then reintroducing them separately to see what effect they have.

Many of the people I've worked with, myself included, found no specific irritants AFTER the elimination. Several went in sure they were at least intolerant of some food(s), and came out pleased to be able to tolerate all foods in moderation.

The time spent on the elimination diet (sans coffee, sugar, wheat, dairy, peanuts, tomatoes, alcohol and chocolate) allowed the stomach to restore its vitality so it was no longer functioning under a state of shock.

Eating Alive II provided me insight into the importance of local fare keeping the sodium/potassium balance in check, which has proved to be a very important factor in the health restorations I have conducted or facilitated.

Hot and Bothered

Dr Matsen's views that trouble begins in the stomach and spreads throughout the body seemed a likely answer to the health problems I saw everyday. He also preached of the dangers of mercury exposure, and its common occurrence in western society; more on this later.

Restoring the seasonal, sun based sodium/potassium balance allows proper vitamin D absorption and distribution which allows proper calcium uptake thus restoring efficiency to the ileocecal valve; another key problem in the digestive dysfunction junction.

When combined with de-shocking the stomach, this restoration project really cranks up people's digestive health which can lead to a new-found wealth of energy and positivity. If left unchecked, the shell shocked stomach and the illin' ileocecal valve create havoc, bacterial overgrowth and spillover, and, you guessed it; inflammation.

Eventually, the inflammation reaches other parts of the body and the effects are varied, dependant on each individual's unique immune response. Once they manifest into symptoms that Doctors can categorize they are clumped together and labeled with odd, Latin, mythical, medical names.

The common denominator is always inflammation, and removing the cause is always the start. I've always appreciated the functional medicine approach and writings of Dr Mark Hyman, especially his *Ultrametabolism*; one of the books that helped me shift into a more holistic health mind frame. Functional medicine is the view that the body's systems are all connected and affect one another's function. This also entails the belief that the body can and will heal itself, given the opportunity and materials needed.

He gives a great analogy that diet or some other source of inflammation is like a tack, and that the tack must be removed rather than masking the pain with drugs.

I really appreciate his opposition to traditional medicine's focus on naming a disease then applying the corresponding drug treatment. Mainstream medical services have you play an enthralling game of "name that disease" and then tell you that you lose, give you a pamphlet on how to die gracefully, then move on to the next contestant. Come on down!

Instead, functional medicine seeks to find the cause of the problem and to treat it through diet and lifestyle choices and high quality food supplements, such as vitamins or minerals. It sure beats the proverbial death sentence modern medicine hands you.

The explanations of elimination of dietary and lifestyle related inflammation fit nearly perfectly with those I'd already been practicing. There were more detailed explanations of cause and effect, as nutrigenomics, the study of how food affects our genes, was a new field at the time. It brought with it great insight into the healing powers of food and the harmful toxicity of fake foods.

The more science I found to support this information, the more I realized science to be confirming the practices of our ancestors. Before humans had the means to prove our practices, the powers of observation we possessed and the ancient wisdom imparted forged our genes, our strengths and weaknesses. They have with stood the tests of time, and now, the tests of modern man.

While your first defense is an abundance of whole foods in harmony with nature and your genes, occasional fasting to allow for spring cleaning, exercise to speed detox and keep you fit, supplementing with sprouts, lots of quality sleep, and a positive mental outlook; there is always more you can do. It will be hard to out-detox the polluters, so every step you take is important.

Improving air and water quality through filtration is an important step, as these are the two most important nutrients to human beings. You can't live more than a few minutes without air, days without water and weeks to months without food.

Every cell and function within our bodies depends on water, so be sure to get plenty of it and take steps to remove its contaminants. Be sure to filter bath and shower water as the heat used turns the chlorine into vapor which is then inhaled.

Choosing organic foods or becoming familiar with local farmers' techniques and deciding for yourself is another great decision to avoid toxicity in your food. Many small farms use organic practices but do not get certified as organic due to the cost. Avoiding processed, boxed foods and buying whole foods, then cooking for yourself is also a great way to limit your exposure to harmful additives and preservatives.

Be wary too, of antiquated "pro health" practices such as vaccinations and the aforementioned chlorine and fluoride, which have essentially been a long term science experiment on the human race. If you had a shot that contains thimerosol, which is a form of the incredibly toxic mercury, as a preservative, you have been an unknowing participant in another of humanity's great self-inflicted experiments.

Many other ingredients in vaccines are dangerous, or at least not yet proven safe, to humans, yet we continue to be told to use them. More and more flu vaccines with crazy names reminiscent of a Star Wars robot are propagated as necessary, yet again a clear indicator of the money over health brigade working its magic.

New names for old strains of virus, fear mongering on every news program, and ease of availability all add up to a business that perpetuates the news, which perpetuates the next new drug or vaccine.

If you're starting to wonder if these companies may be somehow connected, you're starting to get the picture.

Mercury in silver dental fillings is another example of industry over the consumer's health. Your toothpaste, shampoo, conditioner, soap, hair dye, make up and deodorant are all suspect too.

Take a look at their ingredient lists sometime. Hard to read, let alone pronounce or comprehend. The government regulates these industries, however, they do not fully understand what they should be looking for.

No one does; there are far too many chemicals and toxins that we don't even know of, let alone have tested and their safety and long term effects determined. More chemicals are created every day than are tested in a year! Government watchdogs will never be able to keep up, let alone catch up.

Be wary of the toxins you knowingly ingest too; caffeine, dairy, white sugar, white flour, gluten and alcohol all irritate your stomach and therefore your digestive system. Most people would benefit greatly from eliminating the irritating foods from their diet for a few weeks, to allow the stomach to heal and for the spring cleaning to take place. Green tea has much less caffeine than coffee, and it boasts an impressive roster of antioxidants.

White sugar is an empty calorie, devoid of any nutritional value. Instead choose natural sweeteners like maple syrup, honey, molasses or raw cane sugar that in addition to their sweetness, supply you with vitamins, minerals and antioxidants. The key is to seek healthier options and to use only foods with nutritional value.

I recently read a study that not only made my day, it also made me drool. The study was on the beneficial factors in traditional Canadian maple syrup.

Long prized up here because of its incredible sweetness and rich flavour, scientist sought to prove that it was more than just sugary liquid oft imitated but never duplicated by food manufacturers.

And prove it they did! Two brand new, never before seen antioxidants were discovered, as well as some previously known nutrients added to the all-star roster. Suddenly I'm thinking about pancakes and maple syrup, and I'm getting off track. Back to Detox and eliminating foods.

After a period of elimination, try reintroducing the eliminated foods one at a time for a week or more to see if they cause any digestive upset or recurrence of your symptoms.

If it aggravates your body, it is an irritant and you should not consume it – your life could very well depend on it. If you reintroduce more than one food at a time, you'll never know which caused you harm.

Sometimes your body gets too overloaded and although no specific nutrient aggravates it, the sum of all nutrients and other factors can wreak havoc. By taking away this shock to the stomach you may find all the foods you removed to cause no ill symptoms.

After relieving the state of shock, the stomach might be able to handle them all efficiently. If you feel worse, or the symptoms return, you have found an offending food.

Sourdough, and any sprouted grain bread will have little to no gluten, so they're good choices even if you find yourself gluten sensitive. If you find milk products to be an issue it could be lactose or casein. Yogurt contains less lactose than milk, as the probiotic bacteria added feast on the lactose.

Yogurt produced with fruit does not share this benefit, as the bacteria will feed on the more readily available fruit sugar.

Hard Cheeses too have little to no lactose, making them a suitable option; not to mention nearly universally adored. In the end, you'll see which foods are worth keeping in your diet, which cause you harm, and which simply have no place in your pantry.

Eliminating a food or two from your diet is not the end of the world, though for some it could be the end of disease.

Back to the Future

Technology moves a lot faster than health and safety reports, which are still faster than consumer awareness. For example, the FDA could determine Chemical A to be toxic to humans, and order all companies to stop using it.

However, they will agree (after some coercion, some bling and an appletini) to the industry's demand to be given time to remove the offending chemical, to find an alternative, manufacture it and put it on the shelves.

So by the time you hear that bisphenol A is bad for you, the industry already has a replacement on the shelf knowing you'll spend your hard earned money to protect your health.

Never mind the BPA you already ingested, our bad, and pay no attention to the name of the new plastic we're selling you either. It won't be relevant for another 5 years, when reports are released on its toxicity. But by then, we'll have a newer, new product for you to snatch up.

As technology spurred us forward into the convenient future, we've sought out any way to have to work less: cars, trains, elevators, escalators, nail guns and myriad other gadgets to take the work out of a job.

Future fabricated foods provided more calories but fewer nutrients. Less work and more calories do not do a body good. Humankind began to see the effects of modernization, with clogged arteries, strokes and heart attacks.

Medical progress had extended our expected life spans, only to see us succumbing to disease.

Toxins will also seep into your life through the modernized tools in less obvious ways too. Take for example, plastic. It blows me away how much plastic is in the average kitchen.

We know better than to put plastic in the oven, or on the stove, obviously, it'd melt. Yet how many of us stir hot dishes or boiling water with a plastic spatula. Many also put hot foods into plastic containers to serve as leftovers. As in so many human inventions, the long term health implications have yet to be determined, so we are conducting another experiment on our species.

With all the known toxins in most plastics, and those yet to be discovered (or publicized, which is far more important) it is a good idea to step back to a more antiquated kitchen arsenal as well. Ceramics, glass, wood and stainless steel are all alternatives with little to no negative health impact.

I certainly don't remember seeing much if any plastic in the kitchen of my Mennonite grandparents. Though they were new order, and not always dressed to party like its 1799, they still maintain much of their heritage and farm life ethics.

I recall turning an old fashioned ice cream maker for what seemed like an eternity, to get a fresh bowl of ice cream on a hot day. The garden was maintained impeccably out back even though they no longer worked the farm; these folks weren't afraid of putting a little elbow grease into a task.

We should embrace this idea, apply it to everyday life, and learn to provide more for ourselves. I'm not going so far as to say you should raise chickens and a full garden in the yard of your urban dwelling. However, the more we can control our food supply, our environment and our bodies, the faster we as a species will heal.

D.I.Y. Ain't just For Punx

With that in mind, the next time you have a serious craving for chocolate chip cookies, try baking them yourself instead; you'll save money and you can control just what is going into them.

The same principle applies to whatever foods you desire; learn to create the flavours that you crave, using natural wholesome food ingredients and you will soon crave your own creation rather than the commercial imitation to which you were initially drawn.

The human appetite is a funny beast of its own, though it is a learned response, dependent on your recent habits and exposures. When food alternatives, like soy or almond milk, or just healthier foods in general are introduced they are often met with skepticism and distain. However, if said alternatives are the consistent choice for several weeks they become the taste we're used to and therefore crave.

Humans are stubborn creatures of habit, so change is best brought about slowly unless you're the black and white type personalities (like me) in which case cold turkey approaches work consistently well. Even when making radical changes, the ever present wave form will be present as your body tries to catch up to your radical change.

Change is the way out of the mess we've created, so embrace it before change is forced upon you. Small changes in diet, exercise and lifestyle will always be easier to adapt to than major, dramatic changes like those that follow a stroke or diagnosis of diabetes.

Enjoy the freedom now; the freedom to choose how you eat, and which foods are right for you. The government and food industry won't make healthy decisions for you. The best you can hope for is more honest labeling laws, however for this to do any good, we all must pay attention to these labels. Millions of dollars go into the production of these labels, and the inherent research behind them.

Companies have researched and tested what works best to sell more food, and they are inside your head completely. Things that make us feel good about ourselves, like so called health foods labeled as "smart" or "healthy", will sell to the crowd interested in health and fitness. Label the same food as "Old Fashioned" and it appeals to a different consumer segment.

It's just window dressing; selling you what you want, or making you think this product is what you want. What your body wants is natural nutrients, which come from real food and homemade meals, but perhaps you don't feel you have the time or ability in the kitchen.

Or you may be under the impression that these futuristic foods are somehow better for you. I don't blame you, the advertising sure makes it seem that way. If this sounds familiar you're just like millions of others lost in the sea of commercial processed foods and brainwashing advertising.

I was adrift in said sea myself at one point, however I had great memories of watching my mother and grandparents cook, so when I decided to take on the task for my family, it just came naturally. It's as if cooking and baking were in my genes.

When you approach grocery shopping with the knowledge that it's all just about someone else's profit, it can be very enlightening. It's noteworthy that the products with the least amount of nutrition are usually more expensive as well. Cut out processed food for a month and tally your grocery budget; I guarantee you'll be pleased. Not only will you be in better health, feeling it and looking slimmer; you'll be a bit richer because of it too.

If you must resort to processed foods, and at times we all do, read labels and ignore marketing. Avoid the nutrients known to be bad for health; things like hydrogenated anything, nitrates and nitrites. But also be wary of the things you do not recognize.

Many of these additives may be harmless in small doses, however as always we don't have long term proof that their consumption is safe. Be wary of anything your great, great, great, great, great grandparents wouldn't have been exposed to.

Even athletes and those who are highly active or committed exercisers fall victim to the onslaught of marketing genius. The sports and wellness nutrition industries are huge entities with much to be gained from convincing amateur athletes and fitness-minded people that these products are necessary.

The companies that produce the supplements also own the magazines that advertise and convince you to buy them.

The marketing is so slick, even those wise to the industry scams still buy into them from time to time. The claims are just too good to be true, and if you think about it, we know that. We buy these things with the hope of reaching our goal faster, or in gaining an edge in competition.

We buy these things because we see professionals and cover models saying they use them. The marketing makes it seem like humans are just plain broken and without this product, achieving your dream physique, would be impossible.

Once again, they're in your head and they know what makes you tick; and all they really want is your money. Never forget that last line.

Something I believe you will likely never see is a professional athlete doing a promotion for a vegetable. Or the Superbowl half-time show brought to you by........ Rutabaga.

No, industries with millions of dollars buy big time advertising. Rutabaga (or any other) farmers show up at the market weekend after weekend, they have no million dollar lobbyists, paving their way to hell.

So consider why is it that we don't hear much about the importance of fruits, veggies and other natural foods from our doctors, our schools or the talking screen in our living rooms. There is no major marketing lobby for local eating. There are hard working farmers, eking out a living to produce natural foods for those interested.

A chalk board sign indicating the foods currently for sale, and perhaps forbidding Sunday visits, is all the farmer employs to garner business.

There are little profits to go toward television marketing in order to compete with the like of the beef industry (where's the beef?), dairy (got milk?) or eggs (get crackin'). Familiar, similar catch phrases, intended to keep you buying.

Funny little cartoons or toys to draw our kids' attention, and additive-loaded products to keep the tots addicted, right through adolescence, and god willing they should live so long, until they foster tubby lil tots of their own. Vegetable farmers don't buy advertising to convince us to eat our veggies, Mom and Dad are supposed to do that.

Hand Me Downers

What happens when Mom and Dad don't push those fruits, veggies, and wholesome foods somehow, is the early onset of diseases previously exclusive to adults.

We pass not only our genetic material to our kids, but we also pass the habits we show them, the knowledge we impart and the lifestyle we lead. They learn from us when we teach (hopefully) and when we're not even aware of their presence.

This is no more evident than in a toddler like mine, who parrots my every word, mimics my every action, and steals my every snack. That last one isn't relevant, it's just cute as hell. My infant daughter, though not showing such obvious signs of copy cat behaviour, is clearly watching my every move, studying like an actress up for the role of a lifetime. I see her watching, and I immediately try to make sure I'm providing a good example.

What we learned from our parents, we leave behind as our legacy, carried on by our children; from the dawn of man to the end of the future. We don't know what the future will hold, how far technology will push, how much abuse the Earth will withstand or how much the human body will adapt.

As a species, we've only been around for a blink of an eye on the evolutionary time scale. Our genes have not changed much, but it is possible that they will over time.

The prospect that we'll adapt some defense against obesity seems bleak; however, technology providing that breakthrough seems a lot more likely. Whether this will ever happen, or if it could be accomplished safely, only time will tell.

We have to choose for ourselves what our future will look like, and those of us who've procreated have an even larger role in shaping the world to come. Our children learn from our examples in every aspect of life, and nowhere is this more evident than in the nutritional habits of children.

Parents who suffer from depression breed kids prone to get depressed. Nature or Nurture? Doesn't matter. Set the stage for your kids to pioneer the new world order. Teach your offspring the value of health, and show them the way. Your legacy affects their life. After all, you want to be around to enjoy them growing up don't you?

In the present, you only have the control over the amount of activity you undertake, the foods you eat and the way you live your life. Wait for a miracle, and you'll likely be disappointed. Create your own miracle, one positive behavior, and one better day at a time; you'll be amazed. You are human: the most advanced and dominant species that has ever walked the Earth.

You have a mind capable of incredible things. You have a heart capable of love and compassion. You have potential and you have a blueprint to help you reach it. That blueprint is written inside each and every cell in your body: your DNA.

Change is possible and the capacity for it lies in each of us. Whether this is internal, as in your self-worth and confidence, or external, as in a lean figure or healthy hair, the blueprint is in you. It is up to you to unravel the mystery that is you.

Find out who you are, where you came from and how you evolved to who you are now, then decide who you want to be and become that person. The blueprint for how to achieve this follows in part II.

For your heath, the health of the planet and future generations to come, the potential is coded into your very being. The past can show us how to build our future, if we learn from our mistakes.

The human race has fallen from grace, but together we can rise again, if each of us takes responsibility for our bodies and the life that surrounds us all. It begins with you.

You are the predator, the competitor and everything in between.

Waves

This is the part of the book where you jump in; Sink or Swim. It's up to you to become the Predator in the Water and to stop living like prey. Like everything else in this work, I use natural history and evolution to provide solutions to our modern day physiological problems.

Predation on land entails a lot more of a Competitive aspect in that the territory is limited, the prey scarce, and the competition fierce. In the open waters however, the territory is vast and therefore the competition is lessened.

Sharks have struck fear into the hearts of humans since our inception, and they still continue to rule the ocean without dissent. They are the perfect hunting animal, complete with incredible teeth and jaw power and those heartless black eyes. The ability to detect a drop of blood, and a mouth obviously designed for carnage are further examples of the alpha predator status of the shark.

The Tiger Shark's keen eyesight and ability to sense low frequency pressure waves are excellent illustrations of how a Predator uses its natural instincts and the world around them to conquer the ocean. The world around every Predator, land locked or sea faring, is full of clues and data we can use to become more efficient at the task at hand. Consider the sonar waves used for hunting by bats, and the aforementioned sensory stimulation of pressure waves. You can see that waves penetrate every aspect of this planet, not just the surface of the water. Wave forms are simply everywhere.

I chose the theme of waves for this program because it felt inevitable. Everything I studied or researched had some element of variability, nothing was, or is static. Everything has ups and downs, peaks and valleys put another way: Waves. The image of tidal waves, while devastating and horrific, is a blunt reminder of the true power of waves.

Since the wave form shows up in almost every facet of life, it's impossible to deny its importance. Just as everything in the universe employs a wave, everything in life has a yin and yang, an up and down; a wave. Consider that what might be yin today might turn yang by tomorrow. It's no wonder people are so confused by the fat loss and health industries.

Waves vs Equilibrium

Everything in the world operates on waves, and our human bodies are definitely no exception. The circadian rhythm is a one great example of the constant waves our body undergoes to maintain overall balance. The waves of weight gain and loss, overeating and undereating, that naturally fall concurrent with the change in seasons is a great example of a shared seasonal wave between us and Mother Earth.

Notice how in four-season climates, where Winter is cold, most of the yearly festivities that involve lots of calorie dense foods occur in the Fall and Winter months, when our ancestors benefitted from fattening up a bit. Likewise, our fares are lighter and our activity greater during the warm months, where food is much easier to find in the wild.

A key theme in this book is that of balance, or as it is known in the human body, homeostasis. Status Quo I like to say. By this I mean that your body is just peachy keen with things as they are. Your body might be a complete MESS by your own standards, but your body has found a "groove" and is managing the juggling act of maintaining the status quo.

Everything you do to improve your health and body composition also has a drawback, and every effort you make to change (especially changing body composition) will be met with resistance from your body as it seeks out the status quo.

You increase your cardio, and its beneficial effect increases in a wave pattern: more calories burned and adaptations made during the initial phase cause a leveling off followed by a decrease in the aforementioned parameters. Your body has adjusted and restored balance.

You decrease calories, your body reacts and drops a few pounds, experiences a slight leveling off followed by an increase in the calorie balance via either hunger hormones or decreased activity, whether conscious or subconscious. Again, it forms a wave pattern, as the body adapts, finds a groove and then seeks homeostasis.

Given this ever-present wave pattern in human adaptation, we can use this information to our advantage, essentially harnessing the power of the human sea, the ebb and flow of our own tides. You ARE the Predator in the Water, you just don't know it yet.

Disrupting the Status Quo

There are a few constant, never-ending debates in the exercise and nutrition worlds, and they are all quite similar. It comes down to people's desire to promote their way of doing things, whether driven by monetary gain or personal fulfillment. "What works for me, must work for everyone because it's just so great!" This is the mentality that has driven both fitness and nutrition for so bloody long.

When it comes to fitness and nutrition, the fact is that everything CAN work, and almost everything has SOME benefit. However, as your body seeks homeostasis, it adapts to whatever changes you implement, becomes efficient and finds balance once again. Add to this the LARGE degree of personal variability inherent in human physiology, and you can see why any one approach will be limited in scope compared to the vast flexibility of using wave patterns to engage the body in a major change.

Forget black and white thinking for a while; let's just enjoy the millions of shades of grey. Yes, a low carb diet will increase the amount of fat your body uses for fuel. Yes, a high carb, low fat diet can cause fat loss as well. Without a caloric deficit, neither will cause any fat loss.

Consuming fewer calories than you burn, on a consistent, long term basis, is the only proven method of weight loss. Regardless of which foods and nutrients you eat, you CAN lose weight, so long as you eat less than you burn.

So if that is the truth, and it makes little difference which diet style you follow then how do we explain the ridiculous popularity of the many, many diet approaches? Easy. Caloric restriction. Most of the popular fad diets employ a trick to MAKE you restrict calories below what you normally eat.

Remove or restrict an entire nutrient like carbs or fat, and you really limit people's choices of what to eat. Naturally they will eat less, because there is just a limit to how much veggies and lean meat a person can eat without breaking their diet.

There lies fad diets' biggest downfall, in that they are a fad, not something you can adopt for a lifetime. So they are bound to fail if clung to as the only option, or even the best option. This is because, after the initial high of the wave they bring about, you're left riding out the end of the wave right back into the status quo.

Go ahead and prove this to yourself; eat a low carb or low fat diet for a week or two and see how intense your craving for that nutrient gets! Once you get these deprived feelings and the endless cravings these diets produce, it is damn near impossible to resist.

Rather than doggedly applying one single approach until it fails, the waves system cycles through different approaches in both nutrition and exercise (or lack thereof) in order to exploit the body's natural tendency to restore balance. Instead of one solitary approach, waves is every approach, at least to some degree and dependant on you and your goals.

Another example of the misunderstood value of variability can be found in exercise too. Here the debate either focuses on type of exercise, or program design. People from all over the world have lost fat through different forms of exercise.

Some got lean and healthy by doing cardiovascular exercise, which is just a fancy way to say working your heart and lungs. Joe Kegbelly starts running everyday and he loses a bunch of fat.

Lots of people got lean and healthy by resistance training, which just means working against a resistance such as a barbell, a rubber band or gravity. Joe Kegbelly becomes Joe Sixpack by lifting weights to lose fat.

Others still employed NO formal exercise and still lost weight! This just proves that the bottom line is a calorie deficit. So long as there is a caloric deficit created by caloric restriction, physical activity, or both, weight will be lost. So why all the arguments over which method is better? What we're missing here is an analysis of the quality of weight lost, not just quantity.

Strength training has been shown to help maintain muscle mass in the face of a caloric deficit. In fact, study after study has shown that when dieters incorporated resistance training, they lost more fat by preserving their muscle mass! It's the old adage "use it or lose" for REAL!!!

With this info in mind, you can surmise that when folks diet without any strength training, they lose muscle along with fat, which means lower body WEIGHT does NOT necessarily make for a more physically appealing body.

If you weigh less, but also have less calorie-consuming muscle, you are actually worse off in the long term. By building, or at least maintaining your muscles, you keep a higher metabolic rate as those muscles need to be fueled to produce movement.

On the other hand, someone with tons of muscle but who can hardly walk up a flight of stairs due to poor cardiovascular ability isn't any better off really. This is because all the different repetition ranges in weight lifting have different effects, and none is the be all and end all of strength training. High repetition work has more effect on your cardiovascular health than does low rep training.

Low rep work involves neural adaptations far more than high rep training. High rep training depletes glycogen best, which speeds up fat loss. Low rep work causes less muscular fatigue and more systemic fatigue. High rep training induces changes at the cellular level, resulting in increased storage and size, whereas low rep training induces denser muscle growth at the level of muscle fibers.

As I said earlier, everything has its place, and this is very true for fitness and nutrition. High repetition weight lifting works, low rep works, and so does everything in between! As in anything related to the human body, balance will be sought and eventually achieved, when you take on a new style of training, and if you guessed that it too takes on a wave form, well you might just be getting it now!

So high carb diets can cause fat loss, and low carb diets can cause fat loss; high rep training works and so does low rep training. Confused yet?

It's too simple to just look at the net effect of these parameters and make assumptions based on bottom lines only. Rather, the Waves system looks at the details of each approach and how to sidestep the physiological downsides to each one. The Waves Doctrine also looks at how each approach can be fused together in a chain, where the peak of one cycle precedes the beginning of the next.

As mentioned, after a few days of low carb dieting or at least glycogen depletion, your body becomes more efficient at burning body fat as fuel. The Waves system uses high repetition weight lifting and/or cardio to further deplete glycogen to boost this effect even more. Due to limited supply of carbs, and increased supply of dietary fat, your body seeks balance and becomes more efficient at burning fat as fuel (both dietary and body fat).

The same is true of a high carb diet, in that after a few days high carbing, your body shift from being a fat burner to being more of a sugar burner. Unless the dieter is already pretty lean and looking to increase their endurance performance, this has no real use for our purposes, as we'd prefer to stay in the fat burning efficiency mode.

For that reason, Waves starts the carb loading at 24 hours maximum. This gives you about 6 meals eating high carb and no higher than maintenance calories, or even maintaining a small caloric deficit while fat burning is at its peak.

The Waves system employs another workout prior to carb loading to ensure maximum nutrient uptake, which limits the potential for fat storage during overeating. Medium to high repetitions would be the best choice here, or some other form of glycogen draining exercise.

Too Much of a Good Thing

Some folks will find 24 hours too much, and will have to practice discipline by cutting the 24 hours down to the level that works best individually. This might mean striving for smaller amount of carbs, or cutting the 24 hours back.

In order to stay in a caloric deficit while taking in way more carbs than usual, you have to limit the dietary fat you eat. As the high carb day pushes your body back into muscle building, repair and storage (aka Anabolism), you want to limit the fat that can be stored as a side effect.

So we're talking about a low fat, high carb diet with moderate amounts of protein. It can be tough to limit the fat, as this excludes many of the foods people end up craving while dieting; junk foods, or foods high in sugar and fat.

While sugar is a carbohydrate, it is NOT the preferred carbohydrate for the purposes of the Waves system carb loading phase. The reason is that despite being included in the foods we all love, sugar is 50% fructose. Yes, the sugar found in fruit, fructose, is needed in small amounts to refill liver glycogen (which helps to resume anabolism) but any more than the liver's limited storage ability will be turned into fat and stored as such. Not good.

Carbohydrates found in nature as starches are the preferred source to refill muscle glycogen, and since we've spent all week low carbing, fasting, dieting or some combo thereof, these are the carbs we want to consume lots of!

Potatoes, corn, beets, carrots, whole grain bread, pasta, bagels and low fat milk should make up the bulk of your carb load.

True, gorging on candy and ice cream is more fun, but this plan is designed to improve your mind, body and soul, not to make you have fun getting fatter, so suck it up and enjoy the starches you've been avoiding during the depletion phase.

I do advise people to have a few "treats" that don't fit the starchy, natural description above, partly because they'll undoubtedly include sucrose (and therefore fructose) but mostly because they help to keep dieters sane by not restricting "treats" all the time.

Shoot for no more than 10% of your daily carb load calories to come from this "treat".

While you can and maybe even should try to make this a low fat affair, nothing is off limits, so long as it is 10% or less. If it's higher in fat, you'll just have to reduce dietary fat from some of your other meals during the carb load to compensate.

The morning after you start your carb load you should be noticeably leaner than the day before. This happens as a result of the increased glycogen storage pulling water from under the skin. If you don't look or feel leaner, your carb load may have gone awry.

Too much fat or fructose can negatively affect the carb load, as can too many of the right carbs. It depends on HOW glycogen depleted you were going into the carb load.

It is a balancing act, and takes a bit of practice to get just right. Too much depletion and you'll give in to carb temptation before the loading starts, or you'll go completely carb crazy once it does and spoil the effect.

You can use this subjective test to determine how glycogen depleted you are.

Glycogen depletion feels like crap! You feel weak, tired, hungry and unusually moody as there are so few carbs available, which also aid in the production of serotonin aka the “feel good” chemical.

If you can increase your high rep workouts every week and aren’t too sore, you ain’t depleted.

Poor performance in these depletion workouts is not an indicator of muscle loss, or weakness; glycogen depletion impairs performance without a doubt.

If your depletion workouts feel like banging your head off a wall, make you feel nauseous, or just completely dead afterwards, congrats! It sounds like you’re glycogen depleted.

Here too lies some individual variability: how low carb can the person go without ruining their training intensity or totally blowing their diet before the carb load. Some people just can't hack a carb diet, you’ll have to decide for yourself.

After the Party Ends

Once your 24 hours (or less) of carb loading has passed, you just resume a normal diet with caloric restriction. No specific macronutrient plan (high carb, vs high fat), just a regular eating day slightly under maintenance calories. This is because resuming the low carb phase here would hamper the power workout that follows.

Eating all those carbs after being deprived of them sets the stage for a great workout of lifting HEAVY weights (relative to your strength levels), increased growth potential and your strongest day of the week. You should feel STRONG going into this workout and you'll likely perform better than you expect. This power based workout should be a low rep affair, with heavy weights and lots of rest between sets. The goal here is maximal performance of strength, which best maintains muscle mass.

You're going into this workout carb loaded so your muscles have the fuel required for an intense workout, however you should still ensure that you've had a meal 2-3 hours beforehand, and perhaps even a drink of simple carbs and protein (dates and whey is an old standby) to really get you amped up!

The extra sugar and protein in your blood will make you feel stronger, while also bolstering your recovery ability. I'm no stickler about choice of pre and post workout nutrition, as solid food works best for some, liquids for others.

After this workout, another quickly digested meal or drink of simple carbs and protein (just like, or similar to the pre-workout drink) will speed recovery and limit soreness. One final "normal" meal after this and you are back to phase one.

As you're carb loaded, you will be a few pounds heavier thanks to increased glycogen storage, which always has accompanying water weight as each gram of glycogen requires 3-4 grams of water for storage.

This is why people refer to “water weight” loss during low carb diets.

The up and down nature of this type of diet can be frustrating to those who expect linear weight loss. However, by tracking weight only on the final depletion day(your lowest weekly weight) and at the end of the carb load (your highest weekly weight) we can ensure that each week is judged against the prior weeks.

As long as the overall trend is lower compared to previous weeks, weight loss is happening and the Waves system is working just right.

When tracking weight through these fluctuations, you will likely become an expert on YOU. Less weight lost than expected during depletion can usually be explained by increased carb/calorie intake. More weight gained during the carb load either means too many carbs, too much sugar or fat, or all the above.

You will learn your body’s reactions and tolerances, and within a few waves, dial it in perfectly!

Smarter Not Harder

If you're following the above advice to the T, have made a few adjustments toward personalizing the program and still aren't experiencing the fat loss you desire, DO NOT take the conventional advice and automatically assume you need to further cut calories or do more exercise. More exercise or harder exercise is not always better.

Low intensity activity, such as walking and leisurely bicycling can and should be added to the plan wherever possible. This is true especially during a fast, and/or low carb diet. When carbs are low, fat use is high, and low intensity activity relies almost exclusively on fat for fuel.

Many people sneer at walking as part of a fat loss plan, and this is some serious misguided distain. Yes, your grandma looks fly in her Adidas track suit, running shoes and sweat bands, but bear with me, she's on to something.

At this point all the dudes out there are grabbing their crotch like MJ, clinging to their manhood as I compare us men to Granny Speed Walker. Don't worry just yet guys, I'm not bashing your manliness or trying to sensitize you by cranking up your estrogen levels. The point I want to make is this: Old folk are told to walk because it is the easiest form of calorie burning exercise from which to recover. Unless you don't currently walk at all, you likely will feel nothing sore after even an hour long walk. You might be a bit tired, but that's nothing a meal wouldn't take care of.

So what does this have to do with you? Well, if you're reading this it is fairly likely that you want to lose fat. You know from reading up to this point that you MUST create a caloric deficit in order to lose weight, and therefore you know that you are providing your body with less than what it requires to do its "normal" everyday tasks of repair, maintenance and recovery.

So any exercise on a diet is a stressor to your body, as your body struggles to recover on a limited supply of nutrients and calories. Many people create major caloric deficits on a diet, and this can be effective if overall activity is low enough for the individual to recover.

However, eager dieters who create daily 1000 calorie deficits (hardcore dieters) are not known for keeping their activity level low; quite the opposite. Rather than JUST create a 1000 calorie deficit, they create another giant deficit of 1000 calories via ass busting exercise. This approach works, very well, for a few days. After that the exerciser's limited recovery ability will catch up to them, setting up all the symptoms of overtraining, and brining fat loss to a screeching halt.

That is how I'm comparing us all to our geriatric counterparts, like it or lump it. I don't care. You may see yourself as healthy, young and vibrant, but on limited food you're more like your Grandma when it comes to recovery.

Ignore this warning and go completely gung ho on a crash diet + insane activity level; you will crash. HARD.

I know, I've done it hundreds of times, thinking I had the youth and good genes to pull it off. Had I checked my ego at the door with my coat, I'd have made remarkable progress remarkably faster!

The moderate approach may be better for you, if it allows you to remain compliant to the diet and training intensely, all while dropping pounds.

You may find that this approach is too tame and you want to create a bigger splash; heed the warnings of this chapter!

You CAN create a bigger deficit with diet, or with exercise, but NOT WITH BOTH!

Every individual will have their own unique breaking point of where to draw the line, however nearly every dieting person I've worked with fared better with fewer calories and less exercise, rather than increases in activity. This is not the case in an inactive person; a sedentary person will benefit from any increased activity. Water is also wet BTW! Fascinating.

Hard and Fast Rules

This brings us back to the wave pattern, as always. As mentioned, the buck wild, gung ho method of extreme calorie restriction coupled with extreme amounts of exercise works well, albeit briefly.

This is the person who is SUPER dedicated to their diet for a week (or less) and then falls apart. Too much too fast, usually means bound to crash.

However, given that we can invariably predict this breaking of the diet in an almost universal pattern (3-7 days..ish) we should be able to harness this natural reaction and employ it to work for us, instead of against.

In this instance, such a radical approach could be employed for 3-5 days (depending on your tolerance) to kick start a more sustainable, long term plan. If you've tried diets before, done great and then crashed, this method is for you! You can rest easy; it's not just weak willpower sabotaging your previous diet attempts, though it could also be an issue.

No, your entire body fights against you, in an all out upheaval for control, by playing with your hunger hormones until you break. Some people can last a whole week before the crash (maybe with very low activity?) others are ready to eat the whole buffet by 8pm on day 3 (likely those taking extreme measures).

Some weeks may prove to be more or less difficult to hold out the diet phase, and these are usually signs from your body about its current stress level. Theoretically, a week off from regular exercise may enable enhanced recovery, therefore decreasing your need for food, increasing the likelihood of a successful dieting week.

Conversely, a week with disrupted sleep (Teething babies anyone? Macy! Go back to sleep!) could shift the equation in the opposite direction. Less sleep, more cortisol/stress, limited recovery and intense food craving would be a likely list of changes brought about by the lack of sleep.

With that in mind, early morning cardio, while an effective fat burner, could be replaced with an extra hour or two of sleep, especially during hard dieting or exercising phases. If you're so obsessed that you feel guilty sleeping in, soothe your mind with the thought that during sleep you're burning small amounts of fat, while creating the hormonal profile to burn massive amounts of the stuff!

If fasting is employed through the morning, your lunch time activity (cardio, or walking, depending on phase) is still done fasted with all the benefits touted by the "early morning, fasted exercise" advocates. You'll also feel better, having better recovered from yesterday's rigors.

<u>Rage vs The Machine</u>

Ok, sleeping in. Fits nice with the hippyish stuff, kinder, gentler, blah blah blah. Here's some more:

Meditation! Yup, just like the Buddhist monks, sans the orange silk PJs, unless you're into that. We're getting down to the importance of recovery and how limited our recovery ability may be during times of caloric restriction aka dieting. So here comes Cpt Superhippy to the rescue.

I'm a drummer, a football fanatic (former player), a metal head and punk, and a weightlifter; you can likely assume I'm a dude with some anger issues. You wouldn't be wrong. I've always had anger issues, as long as I can remember having anything. My parents got me on the drum kit very early to help diffuse my rage. Football was next, though "flag" football just proved how badly I wanted to run through people.

I live my life this way, still to this day at 31 years old. I am a Mack Truck that will run right through anything in my way. At 31 though, I've learned that my intense approach to life may not always be my best choice, or use of my best asset.

Being a professional working for the local Municipal Government I often have to bite my tongue and suppress my emotions and the same is true as a father of two young girls. Anger, in both or these situations does not bode well for me.

I found that a new, kinder, gentler approach to stress management was needed and so I tried, on and off, many times to incorporate some sort of daily meditation to soothe my soul and to help me deal with my anger appropriately. I quickly gave up and decided that meditation was just not for me.

I'd sit there, cross legged, in the dark, but I'd be fidgeting, or just waiting until it was over. Boredom, restlessness, and lack of fulfillment were the outcome and let's just say I never became adept at meditation. Maybe I should have tried the orange PJs.

Instead I researched meditation, and some of what I found blew my mind. The positive influence on hormonal profiles and stress reduction were incredible! The hormonal "fountain of youth", growth hormone, which is released in several daily "pulses" can be directly increased by proper meditation. Many hear the word "growth" and worry, however GH's fat burning and anti-aging effects should be emphasized in your mind. Considering that the biggest pulse of GH occurs during deep sleep, you can see how this all ties in together.

DHEA which is converted into the sex hormone Testosterone (among tohers) also has similar effects in the body, and increasing its production naturally, can have astounding effects on your body's ability to burn fat, recovery from exercise and to deal with stress. If you're guessing that DHEA and GH are amped up from meditation, you're dead on!

Learning of this while researching meditation made me resolute in finding a way to exploit the benefits of proper meditation. I came across a lot of hippy bulls**t during this research phase and it began to feel like an utter waste of time.

The recommendations for learning to meditate were so remedial, and were all suggestions I'd tried without any success. Most of the recommendations could've been assembled into a pamphlet titled "becoming a Hippy" or at least that's how it all felt to me.

Wearing comfortable clothes, in a dark place, sitting comfortably with some incense just wasn't going to cut it; I have a hard time just sitting still for Christ's sake! I needed something more powerful, like a pill I could swallow to drop me right into deep meditation!

I'm not for or against drugs per se. Some I vehemently despise because of bad personal experiences/addictions, or because they took friends from me far too young.

Others I can see the value in, because they clearly help balance some people out of whack systems. Some drugs can save lives, and some are fun! However, sleeping pills would just knock me out which would not have the same positive effects as meditation promised.

Drugs are Bad, Mmmkay?

Knowing that not all drugs are evil, I did research this avenue somewhat but drugs just didn't seem the right choice, as most mess with normal systems, as they're intended to restore natural balance, not increase one hormone or chemical specifically. What else was left? Well, acid would likely catapult me into psychosis and mushrooms certainly never enhanced my calm, so I sought out a less 60'sish influence.

What I found was being called a digital drug by its critics, and somehow I took that as a positive and got real interested. I knew that today's advanced level of scientific knowledge, specifically biology, would lend us a better technological head start.

Instead I found a technological breakthrough from the 1830's!!! Yeah, so much for new agey high tech stuff. Instead we're left with an antiquated discovery from 180 years ago, though it was never given much attention by the mainstream.

Brain waves have been an area of much interest as their influence is so vast, the implications of their use are absolutely underestimated. The breakthrough was that exposing your brain to two different frequencies could cause your brain to produce a frequency to balance the two opposing frequencies.

This was then determined to be effective at inducing brain wave "states" such as Alpha, Beta, Theta and Delta; each having their own characteristics and therefore implications.

Technologically inducing such a brain wave allows users to specify the type of mental state needed. For our purposes the main state we want to enter is Theta, which is where deep relaxation, mental imagery and meditation occur.

Imbedding these specific brain wave altering frequencies into an audio format creates what is known as Binaural Beats, which is the name given to the 1830's discovery. For our purposes we'll incorporate the daily use of binaural beats designed to induce theta wave brain patterns.

The incense burners, tie dyes, pony tails and Birkenstock sandals aren't needed, Cheech. A pair of stereo headphones and the right audio track will send you diving deep into real meditation and the benefits it entails.

I will admit my own skepticism when first trying these tracks; however I can fully attest to their benefit. My state of internal well being and inner peace are beyond what I'd ever expected to see.

Binaural Beats can be used to induce other brain waves, in order to stimulate each state's characteristics, such as learning or concentration.

For the purposes of the Waves system, the other "state" we need to exploit is that of Delta Waves; which occur during deep sleep. People who have trouble falling, or staying, asleep, will undoubtedly have trouble with recovery and well being.

From A to Zzzzzzz

Using Binaural Beats to induce Theta waves and deep relaxation prior to sleep and then Delta Waves to ensure quick entry into deep, restorative sleep will solve almost any sleep problem. It will also ensure we can exploit all the hormonal benefits of proper sleep, without having to knock off more than 9 hours of sleep.

It is ok if you doze off during the meditation prior to sleep, so long as the headphones stay on. You will not benefit from the tracks playing through headphones on the floor.

Many people find themselves waking earlier in the morning at least initially, when using this strategy. This should be taken as an indicator of success; more recovery is happening in less time!! A self-providing strategy is to then use that extra waking time to complete the day's meditation. If you are waking earlier, you should be feeling rested as well.

While meditating your mind may wander and this is fine, as sometimes the subconscious mind is resolving issues or problem solving. If you can harness your mind power, use the time for positive mental imagery. Picture yourself in the present as having the body you hope to have someday, i.e. your dream physique.

Doing so may seem weird at first, but it enables your brain and subconscious mind to begin to see you in this new light. If your subconscious mind sees you as fat, you will unknowingly live as a fat person. If you see yourself as thin and athletic, you will be guided subconsciously to make the decisions that MAKE a thin, athletic body. It really is all in your head!

As selling a cure to insomnia or stress is all about the money, be sure to do your consumer research before jumping on a specific binaural bandwagon. There are probably a million different makers of binaural beats, so be sure to seek out one that is reputable and designed for meditation and/or sleep problems. A solid money back guarantee is reassuring.

Just like the dealers of traditional "analog" drugs, like pot or alcohol, digital drug pushers are in it for the money, so be wary of slick marketing and out of this world claims.

That sums up the hippy section of peace and love. I have nothing left to say on that topic except that the previously mentioned analog components mentioned could be of benefit to those who just can't chill out and relax.

Slow down, enjoy life; exercise and diet should enhance one's quality of life, not become one's life.

Rabbit Vs Hare

At this point I want to tackle another important point about dieting and strength training, and hints right back to the recommendation for grandma getting jacked. The average gym is limited by the smallest plates they have; therefore the smallest progression in weight possible is typically 5lbs (2 x 2.5lbs).

For 20 year-old College Campus Carl, the usual system of incremental progression of 5lbs minimum is fine. Heck, he's loading an extra 10lbs per side per week (for now)! Those of advanced age and/or dieting, and therefore limited recovery ability, are not likely to be able to accommodate a 5lb increase each workout, if at all!

The instructor or trainer would likely recommend they increase their repetitions instead; however this is a misguided assumption of progression. Often a small increase in weight, perhaps 0.5-2lbs, is actually less of an adjustment for your body than an extra rep. Though this depends on the exerciser's experience, strength level, and exercise poundage, often the better approach is micro-loading.

Both physically and mentally, adding a pound per week to your heavy training day exercises is easier than grinding out more reps. This is also safer for most, as exercise form breaks down fast under conditions of increasing repetitions.

Considering that fat loss occurs far faster than muscle building, and also that we're discussing muscle building in a (temporary) caloric deficit, it should be obvious that trying to pile on weight increases while dropping fat is unlikely, if not destructive.

Some experts declare the maximum amount of SAFE weekly weight loss is 2 lbs for heavier folks, as low as .5 lbs for those who are lean trying to get leaner. These numbers bear a remarkable resemblance to the recommendation given for microloading.

Microloading keeps the poundage progression in weight training small enough to ensure not only adequate recovery, but FULL recovery. The concept comes out of drug free body building, wherein the LACK of steroid use necessitates a slower rate of acclimatization. In case you're wondering why the STANDARD is those who are Juicing, unfortunately that is the state of bodybuilding post 1970. Those who get ripped and muscular without drugs are definitely the minority in that sport, if not in any sport.

Most of the (mis) information prevalent today is based on the training and diet methods of steroid using body builders, which is hilarious, because without the drugs in the first place, these dudes would look as bad as everyone else! Yet we're given the advice to copy their methods, but never told that the secret ingredient is STEROIDS! lol

So for the rest of us, who are genetically average, have jobs, kids, bills and a bloody headache, microloading helps to keep progress moving along. Too many 5 or 10 lbs increases on the barbell results in a crash. Too much too fast, strikes again!

Small incremental progression in exercise poundage fits perfectly along with small decreases in body weight and the issue of recovery while in a caloric deficit.

For genetically average folk like you and I, this is as easy as it's ever going to get. I personally will never use steroids, just as I'd never have cheated during athletic competition. I do not profess to have all the answers about roids, but I do know that they have many health risks and ultimately throw people's bodies out of balance and my interest is in restoring balance.

You're going to have to become comfortable with slow, steady and continual progress. Perhaps a tough pill to swallow, but one that will guarantee success.

Dying to Lose Weight, or Dieting to Lose Weight?

Prolonged dieting is stressful, damaging, discouraging and frankly, not much fun. Therefore, waves of intentional weight gain or at least maintenance should be incorporated to help restore balance. Previously mentioned was the natural tendency of humans to fatten up in the cold winters, and this fits nicely with our intentional weight gain phase.

For this reason, your yearlong training calendar should incorporate at least one wave, indicating periods of intentional weight loss and gain. Even if you are deadset on becoming lean and have no intention of building muscle, take heed!

The bikinis, board shorts and flip flops have been packed away, replaced by wool sweaters, scarves and boots. You're not likely showing off your body as frequently during the next half a year or so, so this is perfect timing to relax a bit on the diet front.

A mental break from deprivation, gaining some weight does not have to mean re-gaining fat. All of the changes you've made in your body are shifting you to an overall state of athleticism and health, so increasing calories per se won't make you fat.

Keep to the same strategies you employed while losing the fat, but with a modest increase in calories and carbs. Try to ensure lean eating to make the weight gained equally lean, aka muscle, which burns calories in its own right. Not only will this help mend your mind and body, it will also facilitate further fat loss once that becomes the primary goal again.

I feel it's worth mentioning that this strategy is a helluva lot more fun at Thanksgiving, Halloween and Christmas, or whichever fall/winter festivities you enjoy.

At the end of your planned gaining phase, you can chart a new wave for the upcoming year dependant on your results during the last wave, and therefore, the next goal you hope to achieve (be in further fat los or something else).

Looking at it as one giant wave, encompassing many smaller waves, one can plan around known festivities wherein overeating is the norm. There is no reason, or room for failure. Every break from the diet is planned, and has a specific function. No longer do you need to feel guilty about breaking your diet. You'll intentionally break it, enjoy the break and get right back at it!

So to chart your own path consider the following waves:

DAILY:

- Maintain your fast through the night, and as long through the day as is comfortable
- Incorporate low to moderate activity during the fasted hours
- Arrange meals with more calories, especially from carbs, eaten before and after training

WEEKLY:

- Match days of caloric maintenance, or surplus, with days of strength training
- Create your largest caloric deficits on days of rest
- Add cardio sparingly, if you cannot create a large enough caloric deficit through diet alone

Monthly:

- Structure Carb loads around any planned social events wherein you would enjoy liberal eating
- Plan carb loads to precede any planned event wherein physique is a concern
- Women may choose to plan carb loads around monthly hormonal fluctuations

Yearly:

- Employ a broad overview to the yearly calendar and mark the big eating occasions

- In a different color mark any occasion where you want to look your best
- In a third color mark any planned rest time

Summary

With these details penciled in, you should already see a few waves forming if you begin a color coded "connect the dots" strategy. Plan around times you want to eat liberally, times you want to look your best and times you just want to take it easy. The Waves system is about harnessing the power of your intrinsic desires, innate tendencies and your stubborn sense of self.

All the factors that sabotage you on a diet can be employed to further your progress, to better yourself, and to achieve a body transformation without fighting yourself every step of the way.

Know thy self first, and then ride the wave.

Nutrient Partitioning for Dummies

At this point I want to review Nutrient Partitioning to ensure you understand its implications, and hopefully are beginning to connect the dots in regards to your own lifestyle or training:

What your body chooses to do with the calories you eat, is the bottom line of nutrient partitioning. We can exert some degree of influence on this process with our lifestyle, training, diet and supplements.

Anabolic Steroids represent the ultimate in nutrient partitioning, in that those who use them can eat ANYTHING and still get leaner with bigger muscles. They're also ridiculously dangerous without a Doctor to administer them (aka Hormone Replacement Therapy). We can mimic this effect though, in perfectly natural and safe ways. Let's look at these options.

Training – by far my favourite, no surprise that it's top of the list at least here. Diabetics are told to exercise to increase their nutrient uptake; cardio and weight training have this effect to different degrees.

When your muscles work moderately to hard, they A) lose their local fuel source (at least somewhat) and B) activate what are known as GLUT-4 receptors.

Glut 4's help shuttle nutrients into the muscles while you're working, making use of any pre-workout nutrition. This process works in the absence of insulin. Everybody has heard of insulin right? Class? Hellooo?

Ok, insulin's main job is storage; nutrients floating around the blood need to get put away. In the diabetic example, they can't use, or don't make insulin, so GLUT-4's are their best hope of getting those nutrients into the right place (MUSCLE not fat, and at very least out of the blood).

So we get to use BOTH insulin and GLUT-4s when we train and then eat. Based on this, exercise should always precede your biggest meal, if not many meals. After a meal, nutrients are floating around, getting stored, or burned if needed before storage. See where this is going?

After a big meal, a fatty meal, or hell, any meal, a moderate walk or cardio session can help ensure no fat gets deposited into fat storage. I already mentioned that taken to the extreme you end up a professional athlete (without the money or career) eat, train, eat, train, eat, train, eat, sleep. Burning off breakfast, then re-fueling and re-burning everything = no storage.

Ok, normal people (unlike myself) don't want to work out every few hours, and some people can't or even shouldn't.

So what else can we do? Both Fasting and Low carb diets increase insulin sensitivity, therefore increasing the amount of nutrients that can be taken into the right places. Both also help the body switch from burning carbs to burning body fat.

This is accomplished by depleting your body's reserves of muscle sugar (glycogen) AKA Glycogen Depletion. Exercise, low carb diet and fasting all work towards this end. On the exercise front, high reps deplete glycogen best for our purposes. Activities like boxing, running, bicycling all do this as well.

Fish oil boosts a process that helps the body use fat for fuel, allowing carbs to go to muscle. Ephedrine, with its erroneous bad reputation also aids in nutrient partitioning by increasing fat burning, thus helping to retain muscle mass while dieting.

The FDA has tarnished this drug's record by vilainizing it in the media due to a few deaths by those abusing it. Not using, ABUSING. If you're interested, just google it. Ephedrine is not very effective without caffeine, however, so be sure to follow the EC recommendations exactly.

Fasting too has this effect. By skipping meals early in the day, your body ends up low on carbs without resorting to a low carb diet. This is a tastier option for sure! However, both can be even more powerful!

Too low carb, and many can't train intensely or can't recover from a hard workout. Nutrient TIMING can help with this, and it's intimately tied into nutrient partitioning.

Nutrient timing just refers to the idea/practice of consuming nutrients when they'll be most beneficial. As mentioned, a low carb diet leaves people drained, and usually not able to train hard (some people are exceptions to this rule). However, consuming the day's ration of carbs right before and after your workout (when they're NEEDED) can side step the lethargy/weakness that some feel while on low carbs.

So let's use me as an example; I try to limit my carbs to 50g, on my diet days. That's NOT much carbs at all. But if I apply nutrient timing and take 20g before my workout with some protein and 30 g afterward (again with protein) that 50 g makes me feel like I'm on a high carb diet, and therefore I can train like a beast.

So low carbing most of the time, with carbs consumed before and after workouts gives the fat burning benefits of low carb, while maintaining training intensity and therefore Progress.

This is known as a Cyclical Ketogenic Diet (CKD); ketogenesis is a physical "state" wherein the body has so little carbs coming in it has to use fat, and a byproduct called Ketones.

The next concept that's needed here is a Cyclical Diet, or carbohydrate cycling. This is also tied to nutrient timing and partitioning. Rather than looking at the small scale, and placing carbs around workouts, we're going to look at the 7 day week and place more calories and specifically carbs on days where your body most needs them!

This should be obvious; on the days you workout, your body needs more nutrients for fuel and building, than it does on days where you rest. Simple? When combined with fasting, you could theoretically fast all day on rest days, and employ nutrient timing/carb cycling, by only eating carbs before and after workouts.

Also important to note: being so low carb, veggies don't count in the carb equation. They're practically free for all.

So long as you're lifting weights, you could fast completely, every 2nd day for months on end, without any worry of starvation or muscle loss. Studies have proven this.

Ok, back to it…..After 2-3 days of low carb dieting/glycogen depletion your body REALLY ramps up fat burning, nutrient sensitivity and all the other parameters of nutrient partitioning. However, when your body has been depleted for TOO long, bad things happen. We'll leave it at that.

In order to avoid those bad things, we need to occasionally "refeed" on carbs to get our muscle stores of glycogen back up, so fat loss can keep happening. After being on a low carb diet for a few solid days, you begin feeling starved and you will crave carbs big time!

So once per week we need a different exercise stimulus that will completely drain that last bit of glycogen thus setting you up for MAXIMAL nutrient uptake; in other words you will be eating more without getting fatter. In fact if you do it right, you actually lean out (visibly!!!) while "overeating".

The key here is to do it right! Lol I've F**ked this up so many times, but eventually MOST will figure it out. Let me explain.

The different kinds of sugars have different goals, once you eat them. I'll save the details, but bottom line: fructose (fruit sugar, ½ of white sugar) goes to liver glycogen first, and starch goes preferentially to muscle glycogen.

While SOME fructose (fruit, candy) is needed to switch the body from fat burning to muscle building, the majority of the carbs should be starch: corn, pasta, bread, oatmeal, rice, cereal, even milk.

BOTTOM LINE: Deplete glycogen to increase fat burning, consume the majority of your carbs around training, eat less on rest days and occasionally increase carb intake to keep the fat burning.

Strength Training Framework

So at VERY least, a dieter should be performing strength training in low to moderate reps, with near maximal weights, in order to maintain their muscle mass and force the loss of fat.

However, this is not to say I think it's the ONLY strength training one should do. As mentioned already, high reps deplete glycogen the BEST and glycogen depletion can enhance or speed up fat loss.

Given that fact, clearly we want to employ this to some degree.

High reps and low reps can be performed in the same workout, in something like a reverse pyramid (start with a heavy weight and rep out, decrease the weight and try for higher reps). However, for optimal fat loss this isn't the only option.

We're going to start with depletion for a few days followed by a moderate rep workout with 24 hour carb refeed and then a day or two later, some sort of heavy training to maintain or increase muscle.

Depletion workouts will be based on high rep work, and they're not usually much fun. Any glycogen depleting exercise can be implemented for this part of the week and multiple modalities of exercise might be best to ensure glycogen depletion occurs in the entire body.

Diet is LOW calorie and LOW carb (as much as possible). Bodyweight training like chin ups, push ups, lunges etc. can be included here if the user so chooses.

Fasting and low intensity activity (like walking) can also be employed here, the more the better so long as you feel recovered from it.

After the depletion comes the moderate rep workout and then the refeed, and it continues on like this. There is no denying my love for my private gym, which is geared toward heavy weights and basic barbell exercises. However, commercial gyms work great for depletion, as the machines make working out on low carbs safer. Going to failure or a rep shy is more likely when you feel no danger.

The moderate rep work can be performed on machines, or with free weights. Common sense and safe practice are a must if using free weights. A power rack or some sort of spotting apparatus enables trainees to push to failure safely.

The key in all the depletion and moderate rep work is to make your sets last 45-60 seconds. Weight and rep count are less important here. Depletion is higher rep and usually faster but try to keep them slow and controlled. The weight used on the moderate rep day will make you go slow automatically.

The heavy workout CANNOT be done with machines. Ok, it could if it HAD to, but I don't recommend it as barbells engage more musculature and therefore have the potential for greater development.

My gym is KING for the heavy workout! Complete with loud music, Converse All stars, knee-high white socks, training belt and sweat band! Yes, performance at the expense of image; but who gives a s**t?!?!?!

The bottom line here is that carb depletion and loading have the potential to create a synergistic system of fat loss and muscle gain without completely depriving oneself of the non-diet foods we all love.

The formula can be adjusted based on individual preference and performance, however pairing low calories/carbs with low intensity, and high calories/carbs with high intensity is a framework that works well for everyone.

Within that framework, high rep work can be used to enhance glycogen depletion (15 x3 or something similar) and to set up the carb load (6-12x2) while heavy weight training (2-3 sets of 2-5) can maintain or even increase lean muscle mass.

Dieting 101

Ok, class is back in session and I hope at this point you have a firm grasp on the info presented thus far, and that you're charged up for the plan, ready to put it to work!

So you know the bottom line is caloric deficit to elicit weight loss. Start here: determine the calorie level that maintains your current weight, for 1-2 weeks.

Do this by using some sort of calorie counter and keep records. Whether it's an app on your iPhone, a web-based program, or an old-fashioned book complete with pencil scribblings, JUST track it! Remember that initially a few pounds of quick loss can be chalked up to water, but that's good!

Next comes some experimentation; determine how low carb and how low calorie you can go while still feeling ok, training hard and most important, not breaking the diet plan. Ideally carbs no lower than 50g/day, no more than 100g on dieting days.

If this is too hard you'll have to find what works for you. Some people swear they just can't do low carb. That's fine, it can be helpful, but it's not 100% necessary. So long as calories are low enough you'll lose weight.

As the diet portion of the initial wave only lasts 4 days or so, a significant cut to calories is ok.

Normally, 10-20% deficit under maintenance is recommended, however in this instance you can cut up to 50% or minimum 1200 calories per day! Hell, some can even break those rules without any detriment!

How low cal is dependent on your threshold for deprivation. I try to eat as little as possible during my depletion phase. Your body will tell you if it needs more, so listen.

However, if you know you're already over your calories, and your body is still telling you to eat, well, it might just be wrong. Willpower is needed here to chisel out that new physique you want; so suck it up and have a glass of water instead.

Cravings are a biotch, but they're also important as they help keep humans alive, and equally important, balanced. Sweat too much and you'll crave meat or salty foods, to replace the sodium. Too hungry, you'll likely crave sweets as your body is desperate to increase its blood glucose. With time, you'll learn to understand the language your body uses to talk to you, and you'll be glad you listened!

Jackasssayswhat?

The problem with this approach is the assumption that people will ever get to a point of understanding with their body's nutritional needs (not desires!).

With the amount of fake foods, additives, preservatives and toxic sheit in our food (and therefore our bodies) the communication lines are fuzzy, to say the least. Disconnected, smashed and burned more accurately describes this dysfunctional relationship between you and your body.

So we need to clear the air, so to speak, by removing all the static noise from your body so the many signals from your various body systems can clearly reach their intended listening audience; you!

The key then is finding the offending noise makers and silencing them once and for all.

Everyone has heard of gluten by this point in time, and many of you have probably tried an elimination diet based on a perceived gluten intolerance. The reason is because mainstream media began talking about how gluten could make you fat and sick without a caloric surplus. People bought this immediately because it places the blame somewhere other than the owner of said fat and sick body. No one wants to be the reason they fail; it feels so much better to blame someone else!

Most gluten free diets caused a few pounds of weight loss, some as high as 10-12 pounds!!! Yep, water; you're really catching on!

When people didn't immediately feel "better" (whatever that means) they would conclude "I guess gluten isn't my problem" and they'd be back to square one.

What they missed is that healing from years of abuse takes time, and on top of that, there may be multiple intolerances present. Removing gluten does nothing if you're also intolerant of dairy, or corn, or caffeine.

WHOA! Back it up, Buckaroo. Caffeine? You mean my standard 22oz Starbucks go to, pick me up? Well maybe.

Let me start out by saying, that if caffeine had an endorsement deal, I would be its posterboy! I LOVE the stuff! Especially as it is found in coffee. MMmmmmm, Mmmmmmm! I'm having one as I write at the moment. So I'm not hating on the stuff. Believe me.

That said, I recognize that caffeine is also a drug. Yes, a drug, specifically an alkaloid, that helps us increase our adrenaline response, even if we're sitting at a computer typing, and not running full steam, trying to kill a boar for dinner. Therein lies the issue: chemical energy when we don't really need it.

To Kill a Walrus or a Waffle?

Do you need increased adrenaline first thing in the morning? Maybe; did a lion wake you up? No? An alarm clock did, gotcha.

The alarm was to wake you for an epic battle for your life, or maybe a competitive event? No, had to get the kids ready for school, understood.

First off, our bodies should produce MORE than enough adrenaline and energy for these tasks and caffeine shouldn't be required to get the day going, or to keep it going, though some low carb days will make it seem this way.

Second, reliance on chemical energy decreases your own ability to produce enough naturally. If you're the type who feels like a zombie before their morning coffee, or can't function until after said brew, you have overworked your adrenal glands.

When overworked, your poor adrenal glands can't produce energy their normal way, or it's just not enough to do the job, since standards are now being met synthetically. Your body may just be immune to caffeine's effects after so much abuse.

Lastly, all this false information and borrowed energy will come back to haunt you with their eventual crash.

They also send out more static noise that your cloud your body's internal lines of communication, thus adding to this growing problem of being out of touch with your body; truly "out of whack".

So a realignment of bodily systems in needed; resetting the inflammatory status quo if you will.

A more comprehensive program of elimination dieting can be implemented to not only root out any intolerances, but to squash the static noise that is impairing communication and function in your body.

Before we get to those details I just want to touch a bit more on the static noise I keep referring to.

Inflammation is a protective response in our bodies, speeding healing of an injury, or creating "markers" for potential muscle growth after exercise, however it can become absolutely destructive if it gets out of control.

The nature of the destruction is specific to the individual, but nearly ALL diseases have a root in inflammation gone awry. By retuning inflammation to a normal baseline, the "acute" spikes caused by stressors (good and bad) will be able to do their job, communicating clearly and authoritatively; in the absence of the static noise, every system in your body is listening and getting the message correct.

No telephone game BS, no typos in gene expression (aka mutation). Just a message, and its reception; Balance.

So who are the usual suspects, implicated in the greatest robbery of all time (the stealing of humankind's good health)? We'll start with gluten and caffeine since we've already identified them publicly.

Gluten is a protein found in wheat (and a few other grains) and nearly every processed food. It is cheap, and does a phenomenal job of helping ingredients stick together in baking, and also provides a nice rich creamy texture. However, inside your body, beyond your taste buds, gluten ain't so sweet no more!

Many people aren't able to properly digest gluten, and this causes all sorts of problems. Saving the gory details, the end result is inflammation as is true of any of the foods we're looking at as being suspicious.

Caffeine too is on the hit list, however due to its overwhelming health benefits and miniscule caffeine content, Green Tea is on the ALLOWED list. Suspect is every other caffeine containing food, beverage or supplement. Your body needs a few weeks to detox from the caffeine dependence we all have.

Dairy is next on the list as there are so many people with problems tolerating dairy. The lactose in dairy isn't the only problem, as many are allergic to casein, a protein found in milk. Milk is also very hard to eliminate as it is found, in some form, in so many commercial foods.

Another food you'll need to avoid, in order to reset the stomach, is baking yeast. Used mostly as a leavening agent to make breads ride, yeast is a close ally and even related to, the yeasts in your digestive system; the very ones we want GONE!

Sourdough rye has no yeast, however it still contains some gluten (although maybe partially digested by the good bacteria it contains), thus eliminating it from the approved list. As for bread choices, sourdough rye, after the elimination, may just be the BEST option for the aforementioned reasons.

Peanuts are a common allergen, and ones we'll remove in this elimination. Any and all peanut containing foods or products should be eliminated. The big problem is actually not the peanut itself; though it can be for the relatively small population who are in fact allergic to the nut. For the average Joe and Jane who don't swell up and die from peanuts, the problem lies within the nut, where there is commonly a mold found thriving.

EWWWW! If that's not enough to turn you off of peanuts, then you my friend, like peanuts a lot more than I do! Yes, peanuts are a common host to the mold Aspergillus flavus, which produces a carcinogen called alfatoxin. Well, in order to render this toxic mold harmless, peanut producers process the heck (and nutrients) out of peanuts, rendering them a natural junk food.

Corn has a problem similar to that of the gluten found in wheat, in that it contains lipid transfer protein. This protein, like gluten, can't be broken down and digested by many individuals, so your body mounts an immune response and attacks the invader, leaving the once picturesque country side battlefield (your insides) a scorched, barren wasteland.

Thankfully not everyone is affected, but this allergy is far more common than people realize and corn is found, as always, in almost every commercial food product.

Some people can have negative reactions to tomatoes, and their products like pizza and pasta sauce, soups or otherwise. Containing a toxic alkaloid, tomatine, before ripening, and in their stems and leaves, tomatoes shouldn't be considered extremely dangerous, as it takes a lot of tomatine to kill you. However, how much it takes to cause problems is unclear. There is also the issue of the acidity of tomatoes and the negative side effects some people experience from overacidity.

Sugar is another culprit whose crimes resemble those already mentioned. However sugar also robs your body of its inherent nutrients. Sugar is an empty calorie, and while in addition to making it easy to get fat, takes nutrients from your body to neutralize it. So not only does it not add any nutrition, it actually takes some away! That's a double whammy in my books!

The only restricted meat are pork and shellfish, and this is they have been found to be or contain common allergens to humans. The fact that many major religions have outlawed, or at least put restrictions on pork and shellfish consumption should be taken as fair warning. There is more to this than the old "pigs are dirty animals" argument.

Alcohol, unfortunately, is also on this list. Sad, I know. Booze can be a lot of fun! It can also be incredibly destructive. Everyone has seen the sorrow of an alcoholic as they battle this horrible “disease” yet few bother to think how it could be negatively affecting the health of those who can consume it in moderation.

Alcohol is a toxin, so when you drink it, your body’s first reaction is something akin to “Get this S**t out of here!” Because alcohol is a toxin, neutralizing it becomes your body’s number one priority, and this produces “byproducts” that can mess with people’s immune system.

Some people flush, some get stuffy or runny noses, some have an unresistable urge to get naked and party like a rockstar! Your genetics likely play a role here, and different ethnicities have been found to have varying levels of reactions to booze.

Being of German and Scottish heritage, I feel fairly confident that booze, at very least Scotch and beer, would have been consumed by my ancestors for a long time! So I’m not too concerned that it might be an issue FOR ME!

However, it does negatively affect your stomach’s ability to talk to the rest of the body. Because of this, and the inflammation/stress it can cause, we’re going to eliminate all forms of alcohol for our elimination.

Allow me to say here, we will reintroduce it, and most people don’t find any trouble with it after the detox. Also it can be included properly in the plan on a weekly basis in conjunction with your carb load, if desired, and no negative reaction is experienced.

This elimination diet is optional (and very effective), will last 2-3 weeks, and you can speed along the elimination by taking probiotic supplements, which will give your gut a good head start on rebuilding. This is a very good idea for those with some underlying health issue in addition to a desired weight loss.

So to sum up: for 2-3 weeks CUT OUT ALL wheat, dairy, caffeine, sugar, yeast, peanuts, corn, tomatoes, pork, shellfish and alcohol. If you smoke, ankle that s**t too. Lol Now is the time; we want to eliminate ALL sources of internal stress/inflammation.

NEXT: for 2-3 more weeks we're going to take advantage of the favourable state your body is in after a RAPID decrease in inflammation/stress. We do this by furthering the stronghold of "good" bacteria in the gut, continuing to take probiotics, but now also adding some sort of a yeast killer, which further weakens the enemy stronghold.

Wild oregano oil, capryllic acid and garlic, are just a few of the yeast killers, and probably the most popular and therefore easy to find. While the elimination diet fertilizes the soil, and the probiotics sow the seed, yeast killers can be viewed as pest control in this analogy. Yeast killers make sure no competing, or destructive organism will be working against your best detox efforts.

The final phase of this program is the planned reintroduction of the offending foods you've now spent 4-6 weeks avoiding. Start by reintroducing ONE food at a time ONLY!!! Adding back more than one will skew the results and mask any true intolerance you were trying to identify.

So add each food back to the diet for 1-2 weeks, and monitor your health, well-being and weight. Any negative reactions should be documented along with the reintroduced food and what else it was consumed with. If when you add dairy back in, and you find it bloats you or sends you right to the bathroom, it likely is an offending food and one of those of which you should be cautious.

There are many more potential allergenic foods, probably as many as there are foods to choose from, however MOST people will benefit greatly from a few weeks of this elimination diet which identifies the usual suspects.

If none of the suspected foods cause problems upon reintroduction, you may not have any intolerance. Rather, it may have been an overall state of an overburdened digestive system.

You should still feel better, digest your food more efficiently and experience less of the negative symptoms with which you began this elimination.

While making you feel better is awesome, and better digestion super, the real key here is that it will be easier for you to lose fat, and you will experience less cravings than before.

You will also become more in touch with your body, therefore better able to recognize the signals it sends out, especially those relaying messages about the effect of a food recently consumed.

Catching the First Wave

Have you spent 2 weeks monitoring your food intake (specifically calories) and body weight? If no, stop reading and get to it! No amount of know-how will work if you don't apply it!

If you answered yes, then let's get down to it! The amount of calories that MAINTAINS your current weight within a few pounds is what we'll call maintenance for now. Next we need to discover how few calories you can handle and how many you really need.

To start you'll need to cut your daily calories by about 500. Skipping 1 normal meal typically accomplishes this. Skipping 24 hours of food (a 24 hour weekly fast) accomplishes about the same as the 500 calorie daily deficit. Either way you go about it, this deficit should cause slow weight loss, maybe 1 lb per week. In those first few weeks it could be significantly more.

If this reduction causes the desired level of weight loss then you're set! Keep at it until I it stops working. If this reduction doesn't cause enough weight loss then you'll need to try a bigger deficit. 16-24 hour fasts on rest days are an excellent strategy, as the lack of activity won't cause much hunger.

I'm more concerned about what you DO eat on workout days, than what you DON'T eat on rest days. Taken to the extreme, you could do complete fasting on off days with no exercise. This could be paired with a protein-dominant diet on cardio/depletion days and high carb/high protein diet on training days.

On the gentler end of the continuum, we'd see smaller calorie deficits up to 1000 calories on rest and depletion days and eating high carb/high protein at maintenance calories on workout days.

Somewhere between is likely where you'll find your groove. Those who can't hack a low carb diet will want to employ the more moderate strategies, whereas a carnivore at heart will have no problem sticking to meat and veggies through the week.

If you can't handle a large cut to your food intake, you'll need to add cardio to increase the amount of fat loss. Keep in mind though, that any increase in activity will cause a desire for increased caloric intake.

So long as your strength training poundages remain the same, if not increasing somewhat, you are maintaining your muscle and don't need to worry about the size of caloric deficit creating problems.

However, if you find you're consistently losing strength, then you are dieting too hard and causing muscle loss. Increase the weekly calorie count slightly and re-evaluate.

More Nitty Gritty

Losing fat and maintaining your muscle mass are the primary concerns. With this in mind, you could conceivably create a large enough caloric deficit from lack of food to eliminate the need for any exercise other than that geared towards maintain your muscle mass. The diet will strip fat off if you remove muscle as a fuel option; this is the major contribution of heavy weight lifting on a diet.

Assuming the dieter in question has not lost ALL their marbles, and is not so completely obsessed with fat loss that they can no longer enjoy food, a pre-carb load depletion workout is rather vital too.

This will limit any potential fat gain during the overeating phase, and will ensure that you are able to perform well during strength training. If you've tried to gain muscle on a diet before (outside of newbie gains) you will truly understand the value of a carb-load prior to strength training.

How long dieting/depletion lasts prior to the overeating/strength training phase is dependent on the individual. Conceptually any size of wave is acceptable as long as its major phase is in line with your goals (i.e. more dieting than overeating if your goal is fat loss).

However, behaviourally, people seem to do better with a weekly carb load, as it provides that short term pay off or reward for a week of successful dieting. If that carb load is limited to 24 hours, this creates a burn ratio of 6:1 (6 days in deficit; 1 day at maintenance) which is as good as we can ask for with a weekly refeed.

Outlined here are the waves that shape a new body, without the negative consequences inherent with single minded diet and exercise approaches. How well each of us reacts to the different approaches, and how long they remain effective will determine the size and shape of the individualized waves.

A daily wave begins the process, following our own circadian rhythm, employing fasting or at least light eating through the day and eating larger, heavier meals later in the day. Another wave crosses one, two or more days, representing the increased calories/carbs associated with strength training and the lower calorie/carb content of rest days.

Depending on individual preference and reactions, the multi-day wave may extend to a week, even two, before rebounding into a peak of higher calories and specifically carbohydrates. Weekly to monthly waves should be indicative of progression in heavy weight lifting and/or weight fluctuations.

With glycogen depletion and carb loading, as much as 15 lbs can be gained or lost without any real permanent change in fat loss, however, if the overall trend continues to drop in pounds and you can at least maintain your current strength, then all is well. You should be looking better, feeling leaner and strong.

At some point, though not for everyone, you may begin to feel as if your dieting efforts have made you too weak. For many this means Summer is over, they've dieted as hard as they can and have stalled. Better than going back to traditional bulking (gaining fat and muscle) would be to employ a week or two of eating at maintenance, or "normally" if you will.

Many find that this break allows their body to recover, and that their fat loss efforts can continue. Even more so if the weights are "maintained" at the current level, or even deloaded (decreased) by 10% and then built back up over a few weeks.

Fine Tuning

Some people will find that once per week is too frequent for carb loads and that perhaps, they never get the fat burning to muscle building ratio right with weekly carb loads. These individuals would be better off planning bi-weekly or monthly refeeds to limit the damage they inflict aka spill over leading to fat regain.

Some lucky people can stay on a dedicated fat loss regime for several months before implementing a refeed. If you can do it, without fat loss slowing/stopping and without complete mental breakdown, then by all means go for it! You'll likely burn through the fat much faster. Most people though, will start experiencing CRAZY strong cravings after several days of dieting, especially the low carb dieting variety.

For the unlucky individuals (i.e. the majority of us) and anyone who is already lean and trying to get REALLY lean, weekly refeeds are likely needed. For the average, it's largely mental in that planning a "cheat" helps keep them on track with the diet plan. For the lean trying to get really lean, in addition to the mental payoff there is a physiological response that is equally important for keeping the fat burning furnace lit.

Another related option, especially for those who can only handle a few days of dieting at a time, or those equally enthusiastic about muscle gain as they are fat loss, is the Every Other Day approach (EOD). In this style, high carb / high calorie days are still paired to strength training and fasting or low calorie/low carb diet tied to rest days.

The physical effect is similar and based on the same physiology, however there is some trade off here which makes this style a good option for short waves, especially following longer waves.

The EOD approach entails lifting weights 2-4 times per week, and eating big on those days, specifically before and after exercise. As an example, if you lift on Monday, Wednesday and

Friday, you would eat high carb at maintenance, and drastically reduce your calories and carbs on Tuesday, Thursday, Saturday and Sunday.

This would create a burn ratio of 4:3. Eating above maintenance on workout days may be necessary for some individuals. This strategy limits the amount of consecutive fat burning days, however, the overall weekly fat burn count is unchanged.

A trade off as usual: without spending a few days low carb, you never fully enter the high efficiency fat burning mode, however you're less likely to overdo the carb refeeds as they occur a few times per week, thus limiting the cravings they can cause.

Given the benefits of the varying rep ranges in strength training, once could conceivably create a weekly wave based on EOD set up.

With that strategy, the highest rep days also entail the highest carb content, tapering off to a moderate carb up after the low rep heavy weight workout. This would be a very advanced strategy, and one not needed for the majority of dieters.

Someone who splurges big time during a weekly carb load could perform their strength training with heavy weights/low reps and a carb-load twice a week, which would shift them to 5:2 burn ratio.

Even though the burn ratio is lower, it would mean for THIS hypothetical individual, a larger caloric deficit by limiting the severity of the carb load(s).

Making Waves

As you can see, you ARE a unique snowflake! You CAN do things your own way and SUCCEED! You absolutely SHOULD listen to your body.

You are capable of determining your OWN needs. You are the ONLY one who can stand in your way. You HAVE the blueprint for success.

Start your wave at 1x per week depletion workout paired with a 1x per week refeed, and 1x per week heavy strength training. Depletion will take up the rest of the week.

If things aren't working right, or if you're not settling into the groove, adjust the waves as described above. This manual outlines many of the available strategies, and especially those I have found particularly beneficial for the majority of trainees.

With your newfound understanding of, and harmony with, the Waves system, you should be capable to designing your own training programs and diets for the rest of your life!

You have the knowledge to review your program and make the changes necessary to achieve your goals. Ride the Wave until you no longer want to surf, baby!

Consider from example two of the different extremes of weekly carb cycling approaches. On the one side is the Every Other Day (EOD) approach wherein workouts every second day are paired with spikes in carbohydrate intake for increased intensity and recovery. In the other end of the spectrum, we have a weekly cycle, with only one heavy workout per week occurring during the weekly carb load. This hypothetical example is based on 350 grams of carbohydrates per week; which *could* also be staged at a standard 50g per day. However, by shifting the majority of your weekly carb allotment into alignment with your more intense training days, fewer carbs are consumed between training, allowing for the burning of body fat. Likewise, the larger carb concentration of this approach allows users to enjoy carbs more liberally, once per week, or more. This enables people to eat normally when they choose (depending on program set up) and also has favourable effects on fat loss hormones (as mentioned previously).

Picture a large calendar comparing monthly to yearly, and daily to weekly waves, so you can visualize the similarities among the various approaches. The major differences are in how long trainees ride each wave. In a daily wave system the waves are short and quite varied, whereas in a monthly wave system the wave form is extended further making weekly training sessions more similar, and at the other end of the spectrum, yearly waves allow more concentration on specific goals and ensures several months of similar training sessions, which most accommodate linear progress.

This is a system of periodization based on changes to loading parameters, and diet to coincide with it. Yet another system could based on seasonal waves of weight gain in the cold months and weight loss preceding the warmer months. Both change on a month to month basis, however the yearly cycle is designed for a longer period, making it more thoroughly planned. The monthly cycle is more flexible and accommodates more whimsical changes. This can be beneficial to flexible trainees and dieters, as it means the plan can be adjusted as one moves through the waves and evaluates each wave's progress.

Also consider the difference in progression between a daily wave and a weekly wave. Though quite similar, the daily wave incorporates heavier lifting sessions, with lighter, recovery based sessions. Often a light, medium, heavy or medium, light, heavy structure is implemented. The daily wave is designed for intermediate trainees, though it can benefit anyone who feels exhaustion from lifting the same weight, or a heavier weight at each successive workout. The key is to go all out on the heavy day, and to take it easier on the light and medium days, though all can be increased weekly.

The weekly wave employs multiple workout sessions based on the same percentage of 1RM, and is therefore best suited to a split routine where each exercise is only performed once per week, and the load increased at each workout. While often prescribed to beginner trainees, this system can work well for anyone able to add resistance every session; this would include post injury, major deloads or trainees returning for some other type of layoff. The key is to increase the load at every workout.

The different systems will appeal to different people, and perhaps even at different points in each individual's training life. You may find that a weekly system is best for you at the moment, but after several months may decide that daily waves would be more appropriate. Unless you test each wavelength, there is no sure way to pick a style. Experimentation and thorough record keeping will help ensure you get it right, and will have significant positive impact on your future wave designs.

Even as a trainee learns the waves system, experiments, documents and observes their progress, there will be times where a new approach is needed to break a plateau. This could be to get into tip top shape for a trip to the beach, a vacation, photo shoot or otherwise. It could also be implemented to bring up a lagging body part such as the arms for men or glutes for women. Lastly these strategies could be employed to break up the monotony of a diet and exercise program; hell some of us just need this kind of good ass kicking once in a while.

Without further adieu, here are the plateau breakers:

Breaking Waves

The following section is of advanced nature, and is intended for periodic, sporadic use, for the purpose of breaking through a training or weight loss plateau. The use of these tactics on a consistent basis will over-train those of average genetics, or cause serious injury. Rather, these waves should be added to the program only after several training waves have been completed, and the trainee has stalled. Once implemented, these breaking waves should only be incorporated for a maximum of three weeks, one exercise at a time.

Heat Wave – Incremental increases in physical demand thus producing more body heat. Here the focus is on making your body work harder while doing the exercises to which you have already adapted. The addition of a weighted vest, ankle and/or wrist weights is a great example; continue your normal cardio routine while pushing harder to maintain the same performance. Sweat suits, sauna suits and neoprene clothing all accomplish this task; however, caution must be used, as this type of training can cause dehydration and overheating.

Shock Wave – Implementation of a radically different training approach, intended to shock the system into further change. Such approaches are intensity generating, not increasing volume or load. Instead these techniques are designed to push trainees past their normal breaking point, albeit only temporarily. Forced reps, negatives only, super slow cadence, drop sets and the like all fit this bill. The purpose could either be to break through a plateau or to specialize on a specific body part.

Seismic Wave – Inclusion of a cycle of heavy singles doubles or triples, with weights nearing 90-100% of your maximum. The purpose here is to determine how your body responds to very heavy loads, and to increase your capacity for handling such loads. Connective tissue and neurological adaptations are required for the body to increase its capacity for handling heavier loads, and occasional inclusion of Seismic Waves will produce such desirable adaptations. Partial movements can also be implemented in the Seismic Wave system to increase loads beyond the trainees' physical capacity. Deadlifts from knee height, or overhead press lock outs are both prime examples.

Following are a few examples of the standard waves implemented by myself and my trainees. This is not meant to be an inclusive list, merely a few good choices from which to start experimenting.

Fat Loss Wave 1 – Weekly Wave

Day 1 -4: diet phase

Low carb if possible and low calorie.

Low intensity cardio and activity

Day 5: Carb Load

High intensity weight training

Full Body routine, medium to high reps, medium weight

Higher carbs and calories – 24 hours.

Day 6: Off Day

No training, no cardio

Normal diet, slight caloric deficit

Day 7: Heavy Training

Heavy weights, low to moderate reps and lots of rest

Power lifting style training on big exercises

Normal diet, slight caloric deficit

Notes: This approach is awesome for those who want to still have liberal eating days while losing fat. Fat regain can be an issue if the carb load is excessive, and fatigue, food cravings and generally becoming a Mr. or Mrs. Cranky pants are typical reactions and draw backs to this approach.

Fat Loss Wave 2 –Every Other Day Wave

Training days:

higher carb and calories, specifically immediately before and after training

lower fat intake + high carbs = smaller carb load every 2nd day

accommodates many different styles of weight lifting i.e. split or full body

Can still incorporate a weekend carb load, by:

Scheduling the most intense training sessions to coincide with the carb loading

using light, medium and heavy training sessions, with the hardest work during the carb load

Rest days:

Low carb and low calorie, higher fat intake

Only low intensity activity

Ideal for fasting, as little energy is expended

Notes: Some prefer to fit an EOD system into a 7 day week. This necessitates an extra day of rest in between two of the training sessions. The "extra" day is somewhat of an anomaly in that it could be a diet day, fasted, or cardio training at maintenance calories, or some combination thereof. Conversely, those with flexible schedules could perform a strict EOD approach, which just means every week's training schedule is varied.

Fat Loss Wave 3 – Cyclical Circadian Wave

AM:

Mornings are spent fasted, with only low intensity activity or cardio

No calories are consumed during this period

Water, tea and coffee (without creamers or sweeteners) are permitted

PM:

One meal is consumed at lunch or later, 2-3 hours prior to training. At least branched Chain Amino Acids should be taken pre-workout.

Training is initiated fed, with some quickly digested carbs and protein prior and/or during

Largest meal of the day follows intense weight lifting

Food is consumed up until bedtime, if desired

Notes: this approach can be exclusively implemented as a fat loss regime, and in many trainees, will produce great results. This approach can also be implemented in conjunction with the above mentioned approaches. Using this system allows fat to be used for fuel throughout the AM, and then food used to rebuild the body in the PM. As most of the recuperation occurs during sleep, this approach ensures calories are available when needed, and absent when not required.

Combining CCD with a sensible weight lifting program and well thought-out pre and post workout nutrition, either carb cycling, nutrient timing or otherwise, is an approach that can be used throughout the year, with only manipulations to training parameters.

All of these approaches can be beneficial at different times in a trainee's weight loss journey, and no one approach is evidently more effective. Rather it is a matter of personal preference, scheduling, trial and error. For many the Weekly Wave is the most effective; but it's also the hardest. Therefore trying to continue to the Weekly Wave will cause overtraining or stalled progress; riding out the end of an old wave.

Instead, when one approach becomes too difficult, monotonous or ineffective, another approach should replace it just as the wave crest begins to level. This ensures a multitude of training parameters are used, boredom is avoided, and progress is virtually never ending.

Now go ahead.

Make Waves.

Bibliography

Training Resources

The Ultimate Diet 2.0 – Lyle McDonald

The Stubborn Fat Solution0 – Lyle McDonald

The Ketogenic Diet0 – Lyle McDonald

Rapid Fat Loss Handbook0 – Lyle McDonald

Combat the Fat – Jeff Anderson

The Warrior Diet – Ori Hofmekler

The Naked Warrior – Pavel Tsatsouline

Power to the People Warrior – Pavel Tsatsouline

Practical Programming for Strength Training – Mark Rippetoe

Starting Strength – Mark Rippetoe

Brawn – Stuart McRobert

Beyond Brawn – Stuart McRobert

The Insider's Tell All Handbook on Weight Training Technique – Stuart McRobert

Nutrition Resources

Eating Alive – Dr John Matsen

Eating Alive II Alive – Dr John Matsen

Ultrametabolism Alive – Dr Mark Hyman

The PH Miracle - Robert O. Young, Shelley Redford Young

12 Steps to Raw Food - Victoria Boutenko

The Gluten Connection - Dr Shari Lieberman

The Thyroid Solution - Ridha Arem

Fit for Life - Harvey Diamond, Marilyn Diamond

Feats that Heal, Fats that Kill - Dr Udo Erasmus

The Metabolic Typing Diet - William Linz Wollcott, Trish Fahey

Cracking the Metabolic Code - James B. Lavalle

The Jungle Effect - Daphne Miller

Survival of the Fittest - Jonathan Kellerman

Survival of the Sickest - Sharon Moalem

Your Inner Fish - Neil Shubin

The Face on Your Plate - Jeffrey Moussaief Masson

The Omnivore's Dilemma - Michael Pollan

In Defense of Food - Michael Pollan

An Apple a Day - Joe Schwarcz

Fast Food Nation - Eric Schlosser

Animal, Vegetable, Miracle - Barbara Kingsolver, Camille Kingsolver, Steven L. Hopp

The Book of Muscle - Lou Schuler, Ian King

The Testosterone Advantage - Lou Schuler, Jeff Volek, Michael Meija, Andy Campbell

Thrive - Brendan Brazier

The Thrive Diet - Brendan Brazier

The Paleo Diet - Loren Cordain

The Paleo Diet for Athletes - Loren Cordain, Joe Friel

The South Beach Diet - Arthur Agatson

DVD Resources

The Blue Planet Series

Walking with Dinosaurs

Walking with Prehistoric Beasts

Walking with Cavemen

Chased by Dinosaurs

Earth

Clash of the Cavemen

Human Evolution series

The Journey of Man

Web Resources

http://leangains.com

http://bodyrecomposition.com

http://www.ncbi.nlm.nih.gov

Made in the USA
Monee, IL
04 November 2026

67378295R00105